# On Leading
# a Clinical
# Department

# On Leading a Clinical Department

## A Guide for Physicians

Harry W. Fritts, Jr., M.D.

Professor and Chair Emeritus
Department of Medicine
State University of New York
Stony Brook

**The Johns Hopkins University Press**
**Baltimore and London**

© 1997 The Johns Hopkins University Press
All rights reserved. Published 1997
Printed in the United States of America on acid-free paper
04 03 02 01 00 99 98 97    5 4 3 2 1

The Johns Hopkins University Press
2715 North Charles Street
Baltimore, Maryland 21218-4319
The Johns Hopkins Press, Ltd., London

ISBN 0-8018-5647-7
ISBN 0-8018-5781-3 (pbk.)

Library of Congress Cataloging-in-Publication Data
will be found at the end of this book.

A catalog record for this book is available from the British Library.

*For Helen*

And for all the students, interns,
and residents who have brought
such pleasure to our lives

# Contents

### III  Solving Problems

### IV  Teaching and Research

# Foreword

It is probably a truism that if you have seen one department of medicine chair you have seen one chair. That has certainly been my experience, and although my tenure as chair overlapped that of Harry Fritts, there were significant differences between my experiences and his. It is equally true that today's department of medicine chair needs to have an agenda very different from the agendas pursued by those of us, like the author and me, who served twenty years ago. We were still learning to manage Medicare and Medicaid, and "managed care" as we know it today was only a gleam in some health economist's eye.

These caveats notwithstanding, there are some universal truths about chairing a department of medicine, and in this remarkably insightful book, Fritts has covered most of them. Moreover, he obviously did a good deal of thinking about what a chair does and how he or she does it. Whether the subject is undergraduate (medical student) education, curriculum construction, house staff training, biomedical research, departmental governance, patient care, community and VA hospital affiliations, departmental relationships with outside organizations, intradepartmental communication, or one of many other topics, the author covers it in a straightforward and easy-to-understand fashion. He also provides some unique insights into the chair's problems and offers some interesting solutions. This should not be too surprising, because each chair brings a different experiential base to his or her job.

This book takes a remarkably humanistic approach to its subject matter. The author, who is obviously widely read, has used Machiavelli's *The Prince* as a model text. Not only that, he has quoted from ancient and modern philosophers, management experts, psychologists, scientists, lawyers, and politicians. One need only note the eclectic nature of the bibliography to appreciate the civility of this book.

Although the author has not been a chair for ten years, he clearly has "kept up" with the present-day health care scene. Managed care is not a foreign concept to him. To be sure, this book does not contain the latest nuances on MSOs (medical service organizations), integrated service networks, or the "for-profit health care sector," but it is sufficiently *au courant* with health care in the late 1990s to teach some useful lessons. Perhaps more important, the book's historical approach tells us that the chair's main occupation consists of human interactions, and most of these have not changed for hundreds of years.

Who should read this book? Certainly the chairs of medicine in U.S. medical schools, but there are only 126 of them (about a quarter of them acting), which is hardly a reason for the book's publication. The readership could be expanded to all medical school chairs, or even to all university chairs; but unlike medical school chairs (particularly in clinical departments), most university chairs serve for short terms and consider the job a burden. Medical school chairs, if they are worth their salt, should serve at least ten, and preferably fifteen, years and exert not only departmental but also institutional leadership. Fritts clearly did both, and he also liked his job—as, indeed, did I. It was the most fun I have ever had (except for being chief resident). But let me suggest that the real readership of this book should consist of the faculty of each department of medicine. Then, it is to be hoped, they would appreciate what a chair does and what a great challenge being a chair is. In this little tome, Dr. Fritts shows us the way.

Robert G. Petersdorf, M.D.
Distinguished Professor of Medicine, University of Washington
Distinguished Physician, VA/Puget Sound Health Care System

# Preface

Many physicians, at one time or another, think they might like to lead a clinical department in a medical school. They know clinical chairs command respect and influence the lives of dozens of people: students, interns, residents, faculty members, and practitioners. Yet, few of these physicians—or, at least, few of the ones I've talked to—know much about the day-to-day work of a clinical chair. A few books and many articles have been written about chairs, but none that I found when I searched the literature covered the decisions, problems, duties, and issues every chair must handle.

This book, written for nonchairs at all levels, talks about these things. It also talks about Niccolò Machiavelli, the controversial genius whose small work, *The Prince*, is the finest guide ever written for the chair of a clinical department, or, for that matter, a chair of anything.

# Acknowledgments

Though I am indebted to dozens of people for their thoughts and insights, I owe a special debt to Gary Provost, my friend and teacher, for his priceless guidance; to Gail Provost Stockwell, my number-one consultant, for her unfailing support; to Dan Fox, whose encouragement kept me going; to Marsh Tenney, who has been my teacher forever and who, thank goodness, continues to educate me; to Wendy Harris, Medical Editor at the Johns Hopkins University Press, who straightened my thoughts as well as my manuscript, and who—if the world and I were fair—would be named coauthor of this book; to Anne Whitmore, manuscript editor, who, with tact and patience, urged me to be precise; to David den-Boer, who, in designing the book, came up with just the right look for the pages; and to the friends and mentors whose company over the years gave me the best possible chance to watch skilled leaders work—André Cournand, Stanley Bradley, Ragnar Granit, Chester Keefer, Marvin Kuschner, Martin Liebowitz, Robert Loeb, Edward Meilman, Leonard Meiselas, Charles Ragan, and Dickinson Richards.

# On Leading
# a Clinical
# Department

# I

## Getting Started

### *1*
### A Portent

On a July morning in 1972 I received a telephone call from Dr. Marvin Kuschner, dean of the new medical school at Stony Brook on Long Island. He asked if I would like to come to Stony Brook and be chair of the Department of Medicine.

The dean had told me about the chairmanship six months earlier. He had also had me visit Stony Brook and talk to members of the search committee over lunch. The job, as they described it, had many attractive features, including the opportunity to shape a new department. Then too, the chair would be working for Marvin Kuschner, a warm, scholarly man and a world-renowned pathologist.

Standing against these inducements were several drawbacks. The biggest was the absence of a university hospital. Blueprints had been drawn but construction not yet started. The second biggest was a reluctance to leave my job as professor of medicine at Columbia University's College of Physicians and Surgeons. I had spent eighteen happy years on the P and S faculty, and I wasn't sure I wanted to trade the secure life of a tenured professor for the risks and uncertainties of a chairmanship.

As things turned out, I didn't have to worry about the decision, because the search committee didn't choose me for the job. Several members disliked the answers I'd given to their questions, so after my visit, the committee looked at other candidates. And as the months went by, I thought less and less about Stony Brook.

Hence, the dean's call in July came as a surprise. "Yes," I told him, "I'd be happy to consider the chairmanship again." And yes, I'd like to tour the new Veterans Administration hospital at Northport, a half-hour drive from Stony Brook. So, on a hot, cloudless afternoon in early August, I met Marv Kuschner and Len Meiselas, the executive associate dean, in Northport. Around two o'clock, we went to the hospital to begin our tour.

Although the construction was finished, the hospital had not yet opened. When we pushed back the heavy front doors, we faced a wall of boxes filled with supplies and equipment. There were few lights in the building and few windows. We moved cautiously, threading our way through make-shift corridors between the crates and boxes.

We inspected the patient-care units, the spaces for departments, the areas where ancillary services would be housed. And all the while we tried to decide whether this hospital could serve as a university hospital until the planned one opened. We talked so long that it was late afternoon when we returned to the front door.

I stepped through the door first, and I was startled. The trees and the grass had a dingy appearance. I turned to the deans and said, "Looks like the end of the world!" Dean Meiselas stepped out, scanned the heavens, then said, "The funny color just means it's going to rain in the morning. It often looks like this when it's going to rain the next day." And Dean Kuschner said, "Out here, Harry, we live so close to the land and the sky and the water we learn to read nature."

Reassured, I thanked them for the tour, got into my car, drove back to New Jersey, and sat down to dinner with my wife. Deciding about the chairmanship, I told her, was going to be terribly difficult.

Then I said, "The darnedest thing. Marv Kuschner and Len Meiselas are straight off the streets of Brooklyn. But out there, they've lived so close to the land and the sky and the water they've learned to read nature. This afternoon, when the whole world

looked dingy, they were able to tell me it just means it's going to
rain in the morning."

My wife looked puzzled. "Surely you know," she said, "that this
afternoon there was an eclipse of the sun."

I did not know. Nor did the deans. But I remembered that people
in ages past thought an eclipse was a miracle, a divine portent written
on the sky. Invoking a portent—even a portent that is opaque and
irrelevant—is as good a way as any to make an impossible decision.
The next week I told the deans I'd take the job.

# 2
# How Clinical Departments
# Are Organized

My first task after being appointed chair was to
decide how to organize the department. And when, in preparation, I
reviewed the structure of departments past and present, I found that
clinical departments, like the principalities Machiavelli studied
(1963, 14–17), have almost all been organized in one of two ways:
(1) with an absolute chair, to whom all members of the department
are answerable, but with a few members serving as consultants who
advise the chair on the operation of the department; or (2) with a
chair and division chiefs, a group of men and women appointed by
the chair to lead subspecialty divisions.

With the first type of organization, the chair has much more
power and authority, for in these departments, the chair is the one
and only leader. If members obey anyone else, it is one of the consultants, whose wishes they follow without feeling any special loyalty
toward the person.

With the second type of organization, part of the chair's authority
is transferred to the chiefs. The chair then supervises the chiefs, and
the chiefs supervise the members of their divisions. This arrange-

ment has the same risks for a clinical chair as it has for all leaders who allow others to share their power.

Robert Loeb, chair of medicine at P and S when I joined the faculty in 1953, preferred the first type. "He detested the idea of divisions," said one of Loeb's senior associates. "He was sure," said another, "that subspecialty units would splinter the department and cause patients to get fragmented care."

So, instead of having chiefs to help him run the department, Loeb relied on a handful of trusted friends. The handful included Dana Atchley, Stanley Bradley, and Franklin Hanger, all distinguished academicians. They did not have titles, nor did they hold formal meetings. Yet, everyone knew that they were Loeb's consultants, that they helped Loeb set policy.

Chester Keefer, chair of medicine at Boston University, where I had trained before coming to P and S, chose the second type of organization. Unlike Loeb, Keefer appointed chiefs. "The secret of building a strong department," Keefer later told me, "is to pick good chiefs, get them started, then leave them alone." And that's what Keefer did. He picked, for example, Robert Wilkins, who would pioneer the drug treatment of hypertension, and who, twenty years later, would succeed Keefer as chair of medicine; Franz Ingelfinger, who would become a renowned clinical investigator and then editor of *The New England Journal of Medicine*; Joseph F. Ross, who would be one of the first to use radioactive isotopes in clinical research, and who would later head the department of nuclear medicine and radiation biology at UCLA; and Louis Weinstein, who would be physician-in-chief of the Haynes Hospital for Infectious Diseases, then professor of medicine at Tufts and Harvard.

Thus, Loeb and Keefer, both brilliant leaders, organized their departments in different ways. Loeb liked the idea of an absolute chair; Keefer liked the idea of a chair with chiefs.

By the time I started pondering the choices, there were other organizational patterns—such as firms and services—to choose from. But I, like Keefer, opted for a chair with chiefs. Implementing the choice was easy, since ours was a new department, without tradition or precedent. Had I been taking over an old department, the implementation could have been harder, for chairs in this position have to decide whether the organization they will inherit should be left alone or changed. If the organization suits them, they will be able to take office with minimal noise and discord. But if they decide to switch from one type to the other, they should make the switch gradually, because few things are more perilous, or more doubtful of success, than an attempt to change the order of things in an old, established department.

# 3
# The Connection between
# Organization and Defense

I knew from firsthand experience that the type of organization made little difference in the routine operation of a department. Members teach, take care of patients, and do research whether the department has an absolute chair or a chair with chiefs. But I also knew, both from observation and from a study of Machiavelli, that the type of organization becomes critically important when a chair is attacked—for example, if a dean decides to fire a chair.

In the first type, the one in which there are no chiefs, a dean will have trouble removing a chair who has made himself sole ruler. The task will be difficult because there are no chiefs to ask for the dean's intervention and no chiefs to lead a revolt against the chair. Then too, the absence of chiefs means that all members of the department are not only equal but dependent on the chair, so it will be difficult to corrupt them.

We have as an example the events in a northeastern school when a dean began to suspect that a chair lacked the ability to do his job. There were no chiefs in the department, so the dean had private talks with a number of department members, trying to get, through subtle questioning, the members' views of the chair's strengths and weaknesses. Few of these people knew the dean well, and most were afraid to speak freely, for fear that their comments would get back to the chair. Then too, the members could speak only for themselves, not for a group, as a chief might have done. Hence, the talks left the dean uncertain about what to do next.

After pondering the matter, the dean asked the chair to resign. The chair refused, then declared that he would not discuss the matter further. This stand-off continued for a number of weeks, weeks during which the department was left in paralyzed disarray. Finally, the president of the university stepped in and fired the chair, a move that embarrassed the dean and weakened his authority.

So if a dean considers getting rid of a chair and the department has no chiefs, the dean will have trouble reading the sentiments of the department and will find it hard to know whether firing the chair will bring applause or rebellion. If on the other hand he succeeds in removing the chair, the dean will have little to fear, apart from treachery by those who remain loyal to the chair. If the dean disarms these, he need not worry about the rest, for none of the members, unlike a chief, has any authority over anyone else. Thus the dean, having had nothing to hope from the department before his victory, will not, at least, have anything to fear while a new chair is being recruited.

The contrary takes place in departments with chiefs, for if the dean wins over some of the chiefs, he will have no trouble enlisting the help of other members, as there are always malcontents who desire a change. The malcontents, emboldened by seeing the chiefs betray the chair, will vilify the chair for something the chair has said or done or published, even when that something is quite harmless. "If you give me six sentences written by the most innocent of men," Cardinal Richelieu had a character in *Mirame* say, "I will find something in them with which to hang him." Using this tactic, malcontents can open the way into the department for the dean and help the dean force the chair out.

But for the dean to control the department thereafter will be difficult, because the chiefs remain, and they will place themselves at the head of new movements, and the dean, not being able to satisfy or weaken them, owing to their number and strength, may be attacked by the department and have his own job threatened.

Reflecting, now, on all these things, we cannot be surprised at the ease with which some deans have had chairs step down or at the difficulties others have encountered in trying to remove chairs. The result, in both instances, has often hinged less on the dean and the chair than on the organization of the department.

Just as chairs are vulnerable to attacks from outside the department, so are they vulnerable to attacks from inside, especially in those departments that have division chiefs. The latter may use their offices to seize power of their own. Members of a division may come to regard their chief with affection and recognize the chief as the one to whom they owe allegiance. Chairs must, therefore, be on continual guard, lest their chiefs become a danger to themselves.

One way to avoid the danger, Machiavelli tells us, is for the chair to carefully follow what the chiefs do and say (103–4), for if the chair can recognize their good and bad works, and can encourage the former and correct the latter, then the chiefs cannot hope to deceive the chair, and he or she stays secure.

The risk of treachery may be lessened in a second way. This way rests on the fact that the insurrections division members instigate are more often aimed at their chief than the chair, and a chair can, if he or she wishes, quietly fuel the rebellions and thus undercut the chief.

But the best way to curb the ambitions of a chief is for the chair to control space, salaries, and appointments in such a way that the chiefs will always be dependent on the chair. This will enable the chair to diminish or increase a chief's resources at any time and thereby weaken or strengthen the chief's position.

Robert Petersdorf, chair emeritus of the Department of Medicine at the University of Washington, has written about the uneasy relation of chairs to chiefs. Dr. Petersdorf reminds us that when a new chair comes to an old department, the chiefs will know more about the place than the new chair does. They may also—through their grants—control most of the resources of the department. These advantages, Petersdorf says, enable chiefs to virtually hold a chair hostage. In addition, chiefs often "do what they please; . . . become masters of the end run to the dean or hospital director; and . . . are members of the departmental team only when it suits them" (1991, 14).

Machiavelli would, I suspect, have heard these words with interest. For when he wrote about the nobles in sixteenth-century principalities who held positions analogous to those of chiefs, he cautioned the prince that, if any nobles purposely avoided being loyal "from notions of ambition, then it is evidence that they think more of their own interests than of yours; and of such men a prince must beware, and look upon them as open enemies, for when adversity comes they will always turn against him and contribute to his ruin" (42).

We can apply these comments to chiefs by saying that when chiefs think more about their divisions than about their departments, and place their own interests above those of all others, they will be a continual threat to the chair and should be fired.

Good chiefs, on the other hand, are a different matter entirely, for they will make themselves the agents of the chair and uphold the chair's authority. They will also handle many of the day-to-day problems that would otherwise be added to the chair's heavy load. And when enemies attack the department, a loyal chief will provide priceless support.

It is, therefore, obvious that a good chief should be honored and rewarded. The chair should treat the chief kindly, pay him or her compliments, and assign the chief responsible tasks, always in such manner that when the chief receives an offer from another school, he or she will not be tempted. Only when a chair and chief stand in this relation to each other do they reap mutual benefits; when it is otherwise, the result is always injurious, for either one or both of them.

From this we draw the general rule, which seldom if ever fails, that a chair who causes a chief to become powerful thereby works his or her own ruin, for the chair will have strengthened the ambition of the chief, who, by either craft or force, will then turn on the chair, and both may lose their jobs.

# 4

# Three Basic Questions and the Means Whereby They Are Posed and Answered

Having decided about the organization of the department and having thought carefully about division chiefs, I next turned to three questions every clinical chair must answer: whether to recruit smart people, whether to encourage the people recruited to express themselves freely, and whether to stay as close to the care of patients as a busy schedule permits.

Some chairs answer the questions quickly. Others wait until they've had experience in the job. No chair can avoid answering the questions, because the chair's actions will reveal what the answers would be, anyway. And these answers, more than those to any other questions, will determine the character of the department and the way the department does its work.

## Whether to Recruit Smart People

The reputation of a chair depends on the people the chair recruits. If the people are competent and faithful, we consider the chair wise, because the chair has recognized the ability of the people and has managed to win their loyalty. But if the people are the reverse, we get a bad impression, because the chair's first mistake has been poor choices.

Five hundred years ago, Machiavelli wrote about the importance of picking good people. He gave as an example the Prince of Siena, who, Machiavelli said, was viewed as "a man of great sagacity," chiefly because he had the wit to recruit the brilliant Antonio di Venafro as his minister. Then Machiavelli talked about recruitment in more general terms. "There are three sorts of intellect: the one understands things by its own quickness of perception; another understands them when explained by someone else; and the third understands them neither by itself nor by the explanation of others. The first is the best, the second very good, and the third useless" (103).

Present-day chairs have to consider two of the three choices: they must decide whether to recruit smart people or people who are not so smart.

Smart people will bring luster to the department. They will contribute novel opinions and fresh ideas. They will also provide brains that the chair can use to keep his own brain sharp. "If I discuss with a strong mind and a stiff jouster," Montaigne tells us, "he presses on my flanks, prods me right and left; his ideas launch mine" (704).

Standing against these advantages are several drawbacks. One is that smart people will ask bothersome questions and insist on having answers. They will expect to be consulted when decisions are made. Dealing with them will require time and patience. They will be difficult to control.

Not-so-smart people will be easier to handle. They will be less interested in decision making and less ready to challenge what the chair does or says. And without any question whatever, they will be easier to lead.

We can fit the foregoing points together in the following way: Smart people will enhance a chair's reputation as a wise and prudent person but diminish the chair's reputation as a leader. Not-so-smart people will bring less renown but will embellish the chair's reputation for leadership, for they will fear the chair, show respect, and obediently follow wherever the chair leads.

## Whether to Encourage Free Speech

During the early weeks in office, a chair should have no other thought so much in mind as what to do about free speech. He or she must decide, as quickly as possible, whether to encourage staff members to speak freely or let them know that the chair will be watching what they say. The decision will always be difficult, but especially so if the chair consults other department heads. Some will say that free speech is a force for evil, while others will say it is a source of strength.

A chair must also remember that free speech is tied to another critical matter, namely, the department's pot of energy. In fact, free speech and energy are so tightly connected that in deciding how to handle the first, the chair decides how to handle the second.

To gain perspective before making the decision, a chair should reflect on the way clinical chairs operated in the past. In the first half of this century, open discussions of departmental affairs were virtually unknown. Chairs held department meetings, but the agendas were carefully regulated, against the possibility that a stray remark would fuel insurrection or erode the chair's control. The real business of the department was carried on in private, between the chair and a handful of trusted friends. A chair didn't need advice from ordinary faculty members. Gods didn't consult mortals, nor kings, commoners.

In those days many clinical chairs were autocrats. They believed in Aesop's maxim that familiarity breeds contempt. To avoid this dreaded pitfall, they stayed above the tumult of day-to-day activities. They remained remote and unapproachable. They wanted to be feared.

The autocratic style suited clinical chairs because they did not have to worry about the goodwill of their staffs. Their jobs were safe, their futures certain, regardless of the way they did their work. A chair of medicine inherited, Paul Beeson tells us, "some more or less 'inalienable rights.' First was the expectation that the appointee could keep the job until retirement. . . . Second, his decisions and actions on such matters as allocation of space, appointment of faculty and junior staff, and division of the departmental budget [would be] . . . accepted with little question" (1975, 73). And although Dr. Beeson was talking about chairs of medicine, all clinical chairs enjoyed these rights and privileges. Back then, departments were small and loosely organized, with a handful of faculty members and a scattering of clerks. It was easy for a chair—even an aloof one—to keep up with what was going on.

But when, in the 1940s, the federal government began to pour money into medical research and training, clinical departments started to grow. A typical department of medicine or surgery soon had more than a hundred members, and its budget, previously nominal, reached seven or eight figures. At the same time, this growth brought an unthinkable development: a chair's performance became subject to review. The idea was as distasteful as it was revolutionary. How could a clinical chair be evaluated? Who would be qualified to do such a thing?

While these and other absurdities were being denounced and lamented, a new type of chair appeared. The new chair—more a liberal than an autocrat—mingled with the faculty and listened to their talk. Isolation, these chairs said, deprived them of crucial information, about worries, conflicts, triumphs, and morale. They compared an aloof chair to a blind person, surrounded by activities the person could not see, much less control or modulate. And the new chairs, in holding this belief, had good people on their side.

Alan Barth, for example, weighed the risks and benefits of encouraging free speech, then said, "Free men—if they exercise their freedom—have a means of correcting their mistakes. But if they suppress dissent by calling it disloyal, they rob themselves of their greatest asset" (1984, 57–58). And Peter Drucker pointed out that "if you ask for disagreement openly, it gives people the feeling they have been heard" (1990, 126).

Such benefits, liberal chairs believe, justify their policy of encouraging people to speak freely. They also believe that free speech keeps chairs in contact with one of their most precious possessions, namely, the collective energy of their staffs. Their debates, complaints, and arguments are external manifestations of the department's internal energy, its latent power, its potential for success. The energy that fuels speaking out and criticizing is the same energy that produces progress.

So if today we look around us, we see that some chairs are autocrats, some liberals. Autocrats control speech and energy tightly. They think a noisy department lacks discipline. Liberals, in contrast, apply enough control to prevent chaos but little beyond that. They think debates and arguments keep the pot of energy boiling. They say a quiet department is dead.

## Whether to Stay Close to the Care of Patients

Clinical chairs should stay as close to the care of patients as their busy schedules permit, for their performance at the bedside will determine the respect paid them by colleagues at all levels. I learned this by watching Chester Keefer and Robert Loeb, two superb clinicians, teach at the bedside and by hearing scornful comments about chairs who seldom got near a patient's bed.

Chairs of surgery, for instance, owe their interns and residents the opportunity to operate with them, and chairs of pediatrics owe their young people the opportunity to help them manage patients. The chairs need not be the best clinicians in their departments nor the ones colleagues always call for consultations. The chairs need only be known as people who give the care of patients high priority. This priority will be evident if the chairs see patients regularly, discuss them with colleagues, follow the literature, and take night-call at least once a month.

In the past, seeing patients was easy. Now, it's often hard. A modern-day chair, Beeson says, "is insulated from direct contact with patients by layers of subspecialist authorities in the department, by their clinical fellows, and by the hierarchical house-staff establishment" (1986, 93–94). But contact with patients is so important that a chair must find ways to shove the roadblocks aside.

Once a chair has fixed the time to be spent with patients, he or she should decide how many hours can be freed for research, for if a chair can stay active in the laboratory, as well as at the bedside, that chair will, without question, be pre-eminent. But if the time required for other duties forces a chair to choose between the laboratory and the bedside, the choice should be the bedside.

# 5
# Government and Bylaws

Departmental governments can be divided into two basic types. The first is found in departments with autocratic chairs. Here, government is usually rudimentary, because government and the chair are one and the same thing. Life for a department member is simple and uncomplicated: the member listens to the chair, then does what the chair says.

The second type of government, found in departments with liberal chairs, is altogether different. In these departments, bylaws often spell out the contract between the leader and the led. Such bylaws require much thought and planning, for even after they have been put in place and temporarily forgotten, their spirit affects the way the department runs.

Bylaws, older friends have told me, were seldom seen in academic units before the 1960s, when universities across the country erupted in turmoil and violence. Students demanded a role in government, and shortly afterward, faculty members joined them.

Mario Savio, an articulate, 22-year-old philosophy major at Berkeley, stated the case for students on the Berkeley campus and, in doing this, spoke for students countrywide. The Berkeley administration, Savio said, paid more attention to the needs of corporations and the federal government than to the needs of the campus community. The corporations and government wanted universities to do research (often, war research) and paid universities handsomely to do it. Savio said this was wrong: "The business of the university is teaching and learning. Only people engaged in it—the students and teachers—are competent to decide how it should be done." Then, to drive his points home, Savio declared, "Those who should give orders—the faculty and students—take orders, and those who should tend to keeping the sidewalks clean, to seeing that we have enough classrooms—the administration—give orders" (Haskins and Benson 1988, 55–56).

Such assaults on tradition shook the foundations of universities everywhere. And in fending off the assaults, many university leaders responded by appointing committees to draft bylaws, which, when finished, were submitted to their faculties. A typical faculty then held a series of meetings, consuming hundreds of faculty hours, in which the faculty, with its student representatives, argued over every suggestion the committee had made. Most of the arguments centered on rights and privileges—as, for example, who was entitled to vote when. But at a deeper level, the goal was to lay down rules that would protect students and faculty from autocratic leaders, leaders who just might make decisions without consulting them.

Eventually, the ferment reached departments, including those in medical schools. For clinical departments, the development was timely, because it coincided with a push to train more generalists, a push that had led schools to add community hospitals as affiliates. Faculties of affiliates, chronically plagued by the feeling of being stepchildren, wanted to know their rights and privileges. A set of bylaws, hammered out with all parties represented, was usually the best way to meet this need. So, in a short time, many clinical departments had bylaws. And it is, I think, safe to say that many departments with liberal chairs continue to have bylaws today.

For department members, the most important feature of bylaws is access to at least one forum where members can express their views. The forum may be a meeting of the entire department, of an executive committee, of division chiefs, or of some other group. Whatever the gathering, it must provide an opportunity for the member to discuss departmental business in a body that meets regularly. "Every student, intern, resident, and faculty member needs a forum," remarked Dr. Alfred Grokoest, a fellow professor of medicine at P and S when the unrest of the 1960s was at its height. "Everyone deserves a chance to be heard."

A second feature of bylaws that has importance for department members is a process whereby the bylaws can be amended. The steps should be clear and unambiguous; they should enable any department member, no matter how junior, to start the process going.

In short, a member of a department looks to bylaws for two guarantees. The first is access to a forum, and the second is the right to propose amendments. These assurances, taken together, constitute the member's bill of rights.

Chairs, too, need bylaws, chiefly for the forums they mandate. Chairs use the forums for many purposes—to solve problems, of course, but mostly to set policy, to fashion statements that both point toward goals and serve as guides for reaching them. A chair does this by introducing a problem that needs attention— for example, attendance at department meetings—and then inviting discussion of it.

Reflecting on this process, a former chair in a northeastern school, a man who regularly used an executive committee as a forum for setting policy, told me he believed there were three tricks to making the process work. The first was to present the problem in precise terms. This meant writing it down before the meeting, then polishing the draft until its meaning was crystal clear. "When I later introduced the problem to the committee, I wrote the polished version on the blackboard, then invited members of the committee to propose policies to cover it. More often than not, I framed the problem as a question—as, for example, 'How can we increase attendance at department meetings?' "

He used his second trick after the discussion had gotten under way. He would take a proposal someone put forward, a proposal that sounded sensible, and write it on the blackboard too. "Putting it on the blackboard," he said, "converted the proposal into a concrete target for the group to shoot at. It also shifted the focus onto the proposal, and away from the person who suggested it."

The third trick was to stay near the blackboard and, as the group criticized the proposal, edit the written draft. "I kept making changes until we had a proposal acceptable to most members of the group. Usually," he said, "no one was completely satisfied with the final version, and at that point I would repeat the old axiom that the test of a good compromise is that it leaves everyone unhappy. Or I would remind them that if a decision is important, it will invariably be controversial."

On a subsequent day, the chair would bring the proposed policy to the entire department for comments. He would also tell the department, in explicit terms, how he planned to implement the policy. For he had learned that a new policy must be put in place with care. Even the most well-intentioned, seemingly innocuous policy can have unintended consequences. And a bad policy, once loosed, can have effects that may or may not be reversible. Alan Barth spoke about implementing policies at the 1951 meeting of the American Association of University Professors. "Dictators," Barth said, "may carry policy into practice more swiftly than governments dependent upon the consent of the governed, but this may mean no more than that they can more swiftly translate errors into national disasters" (57–58).

Foreign policy expert George Kennan used a process similar to the one just described when he helped set policy for the Marshall Plan. Kennan, Irving Janis tells us, made it clear to members of the planning group that they were expected to criticize every part of the plan. "Everyone was urged to express any idea that might embody a useful proposal," Janis says, "and to help spell out all the drawbacks as well as the good consequences. One of the main group norms was to subject everyone's ideas to thorough criticism." Kennan said, "They put me personally over the bumps, to drive whole series of clichés and oversimplifications out of my head, to spare me no complications" (Janis 1972, 175).

Like Kennan, liberal chairs use the young people around them to help set policy and to help keep their thinking straight. A chair who has recruited talented people will be surrounded by men and women with ideas worth hearing. Each person, in one way or another, will be smarter than the chair, and most will be sure they could run the department better than the chair does.

In addition to the points already mentioned, another feature of government bears remembering. It is that all governments, at one time or another, trigger conflict. Moreover, most forms of government won't work well without it. "I hold . . . that a little rebellion now and then," Thomas Jefferson wrote James Madison, "is a good thing, and as necessary in the political world as storms in the physical" (Bartlett 1986, 471). Conflict keeps governments strong.

Elmer Davis spoke about conflict and government in his book, *But We Were Born Free*: "This nation was conceived in liberty and dedicated to the principle—among others—that honest men may honestly disagree; that if they all say what they think, a majority of the people will be able to distinguish truth from error; that in the competition in the market place of ideas, the sounder ideas will in the long run win out" (1954, 114).

# 6
# Affiliates

Before discussing affiliates, I need to speak to our habit of using the word *department* in several ways. We say "the department" when we talk about the department at the school and also when we speak of the school and affiliated departments as an organized whole. Such ambiguity can derail a reader, and to keep this from happening I will use *department*, unmodified, when I talk about the combined home and affiliated departments and *home department* or *affiliated department* when referring to the individual units.

Now, to affiliates. I mentioned earlier that bylaws are important to them. An equally important matter centers on the two schemes commonly used to connect affiliates to their schools. In the first scheme, the school and its hospital sit in the center of a circle, while the affiliates sit on the circle as satellites. In the second scheme, one or more affiliates sit on an inner circle with the school and its hospital, while the remaining affiliates sit on a larger circle, as satellites of the inner group.

The first scheme was the one used at P and S when I was in the department of medicine there. The medical school and Presbyterian Hospital sat in the center of the circle and constituted the seat of power. Affiliated hospitals—as satellites—played secondary roles.

Dr. Robert Loeb, chair of medicine in those days, visited each affiliate regularly—to make rounds, to talk to the faculty, to let the people know he was interested in them. But Loeb, a master of the subtleties of leadership, never let anyone forget the pre-eminence of the home base. When, for instance, he visited Bellevue Hospital, he would say, "At the Heights, we believe . . . " or "In recent months, we've seen two such patients at the Heights." P and S and Presbyterian Hospital were, in fact, located in Washington Heights, a neighborhood on the upper west side of Manhattan. But by dropping "Washington," Loeb made "the Heights" sound like Delphi.

The arrangement at P and S was, with few exceptions, the one used around the country. At each place, the school and university hospital occupied a central, all-powerful position.

When I arrived at Stony Brook, there was no university hospital to pair with the school in the center of the circle. Nor would there be a hospital for the next seven years. As a consequence, our new home department, with its handful of members, had to depend on the faculties of affiliated departments to do all the things the faculty at the school would customarily do.

People at the affiliates gave lectures, trained clerks, and offered electives. They did these jobs so well that we were forced to think about the relation of the affiliates to the home base in a new way. This led those of us in medicine to choose the second scheme, the one where other hospitals sit on an inner circle with the school.

Having made this decision, we divided the hospitals into two groups. The first contained the three hospitals with residency programs. Dr. Edmund Pellegrino, vice president for health affairs and founding father of the Health Sciences Center, had already designated these hospitals "clinical campuses." So we placed the departments of medicine at the clinical campuses on a circle with the department at the school. We called the remaining hospitals "teaching hospitals," and put their departments on a second circle, outside the first.

Once we had agreed on this pattern of organization, we wrote bylaws that conformed to it (see Appendix). The bylaws called for an executive committee made up of representatives from each institution. The departments at all clinical campuses, including the one at the school, had the same number of representatives. In a similar way, departments at each teaching hospital had the same number of representatives, but fewer than those at the clinical campuses. Every appointment, every promotion, every policy that affected the entire department had to be approved by the executive committee. We held meetings once a month, at one of the clinical campuses. We moved from campus to campus and then, after completing the cycle, started over again.

We expected to run into rough spots using this organizational scheme, and we did run into them, mostly because none of us had had experience with a system in which other departments sat on a circle with the department at the school. The people who had the most trouble were division chiefs recruited to the department at the university. These young people had come from places where the chiefs at the school outranked their counterparts at other hospitals, and our newly recruited chiefs had expected to enjoy the same privilege at Stony Brook.

"My friends around the country," one chief said, "can't understand why I don't get to pick the chiefs in my specialty at the other places. Then too, I'm always afraid that the chiefs at the other hospitals are going to embarrass me." So we had to explain repeatedly that our organization was different. One by one, the chiefs came to understand.

When, after seven years, the university hospital opened, we could have switched from the second scheme to the first, because we at last had a hospital we could link to the school in the center of the circle. But the second scheme had worked wonderfully well for us. There was no reason to change. So the department at the school, with its new university hospital, continued to sit on the inner circle with the departments at the other clinical campuses. The home base stayed a clinical campus, just as it had been before.

We can put the foregoing points together in this way: All clinical chairs must decide about the relation of the affiliated departments to the department at the school. A chair can opt for the first scheme, the traditional arrangement for affiliates, where the home base has supreme authority, or for the second scheme, in which one or more affiliates are equal partners with the department at the school. Each scheme has credits and debits. The important point is that either scheme—with a little tinkering—can be made to work.

# II

## Leading and Managing

### 7
### The Two Parts of a Chair's Job

"Being president of a university," wrote A. Bartlett Giamatti, president of Yale, means holding "a mid-nineteenth-century ecclesiastical position on top of a late-twentieth-century corporation" (1988, 17). With this vivid epigram, Giamatti shows us why a president's job is hard. It's hard because it has two parts and the parts often clash.

And so it is with the job of a clinical chair. In supervising things like teaching and research, a chair serves as academic leader. In supervising things like practice income, a chair manages money. Hence, a clinical chair, like the president of a university, sits on top of two enterprises, one devoted to education and research and the other devoted to business.

The business part was grafted onto the chair's job in the 1950s and 1960s when clinical departments decided to raise salaries (see section 9, below). To be able to do this, chairs had to see to it that staff members filled beds and did procedures, two undertakings that propelled clinical departments into the world of income, losses, and balance sheets. Academic physicians began to compete with community physicians for patients and to organize programs to outshine those in nearby hospitals. They also let their parent hospitals advertise the services they offered, thus shattering the tradition that patients seek physicians, not the other way round. And while these things were taking place, the appearance of clinical departments changed. New offices—offices that housed practice managers, accountants, and tax advisors—were added to the standard assortment of faculty cubbyholes, laboratories, and conference rooms. Clinical chairs became responsible for a completely new group of people, men and women who handled clinical income and practice plans. And so it came to pass that in addition to their scholarly activities chairs had to keep their eyes on the bottom line. The following comment by Giamatti became equally applicable to clinical departments: "a college or university [should be] an institution where financial incentives to excellence are absent, where the product line is not a unit or an object but rather a value-laden and lifelong process; where the goal of the enterprise is not growth or market share but intellectual excellence" (36).

The financial incentives to excellence that Giamatti frowned on are, for a modern-day department, the dollars that come from faculty practice. And even when these dollars are a big piece of a department's income, they are nevertheless the sorts of incentives that Giamatti deplored.

Then too, the clinical chairs who must keep track of the dollars have, in most instances, had little if any formal training in business or management. In fact, the norms and habits physicians pick up in their premedical, medical, and postgraduate medical training are said to be the antithesis of those a manager needs. As Michael E. Kurtz, a member of the faculty of the American College of Physician Executives, wrote in a report entitled "The Dual Role Dilemma" (1992, 12), there is "a long list of differences between effective clinicians and effective managers. . . . When factored to determine those that are most critical, a list of nine major differences emerges":*

---

*Table reprinted by permission of the American College of Healthcare Executives and the Health Administration Press.

| *Clinicians* | *Managers* |
| --- | --- |
| Doers | Planners, designers |
| 1:1 interactions | 1:N interactions |
| Reactive personalities | Proactive personalities |
| Require immediate gratification | Accept delayed gratification |
| Deciders | Delegators |
| Value autonomy | Value collaboration |
| Independent | Participative |
| Patient advocates | Organization advocates |
| Identify with profession | Identify with organization |

I think Kurtz got the characterizations just about right. Yet, there is no reason to believe that a clinician, trained to deal with patients on a one-to-one basis, cannot, when called upon, deal with nonpatients in larger groups.

It is also important to keep in mind that the two types depicted in the lists deal with different kinds of people. The clinician handles academicians; the manager works with business people. I don't know how academics would respond to a business-type manager; but I do know that academics, down deep, dislike the idea of being managed by anybody, even a manager who is one of their own.

Despite the real and perceived shortcomings that a clinician brings to the job of department chair, the colleagues I've talked to over the years have told me that they learned the managerial part in the same way they learned the other parts—they got help.

## Where to Get Help

### Books and Journals

Of the hundreds of books that have been written on the management of for-profit and nonprofit organizations, those by Peter

Drucker (1966, 1990) were, for me, especially helpful, because Drucker writes in an informal, commonsense way. The same is true of the old book by Given (1964), entitled *How to Manage People: The Applied Psychology of Handling Human Problems in Business*. Also, books by W. Edwards Deming (1982) or about him (Walton 1986) make good reading, because Deming, a noted management consultant, focused on building excellence into organizations.

These days, a chair can also learn about management by reading medical journals, for in recent years these journals have frequently published articles on management and related topics. Some of the articles, such as the pioneering paper by Robert M. Heyssel and his colleagues (1984) on making physicians responsible for the cost of the care they deliver, are essential reading.

*Meetings*

Meetings of societies, like the Association of Professors of Medicine, often feature discussions of topics that pertain to management—HMOs, Medicare, the relation of medical schools to Veterans Administration hospitals. In addition, panels at national meetings of the American Association of Medical Colleges (AAMC) or of medical specialties are now often devoted to one or another aspect of management. Actually, the most consistent benefit I derived from such meetings was the opportunity to talk to other chairs. I regularly consulted a half-dozen friends about handling practice income, setting salaries, and other such things.

The most important meeting for a clinical chair, in my view, is the Executive Development Seminar for deans and department chairs offered each year by the AAMC. I attended the seminar when it was held in Houston in 1977, and for a week, thirty of us spent mornings, afternoons, and evenings in sessions devoted to one or another aspect of management. Our teachers came from the Harvard Business School and the Sloan School of Management at MIT. The lectures and discussions were superb. And when I recently looked at the program for the 1995 seminar, I saw that the AAMC has kept the curriculum updated. One of the big parts of the 1995 program centered on reimbursement and related financial matters, topics that were little discussed in 1977.

### Nonmedical Managerial Staff Members

No matter how many books and articles on management a chair has read or how many meetings he or she has attended, the chair will need help from nonmedical people with special managerial training, like those who know how to handle practice plans. But I shall delay a discussion of these people until we talk about money (in section 14).

It is a good idea to keep the managerial part of a chair's job in perspective. This part is inarguably important, yet a chair who is a skilled manager will, I'm afraid, be deemed a failure by members of his or her department unless the chair holds their respect as a teacher, investigator, or clinician. The values that faculty members cherish came from the pre-business era of clinical departments, a time in which the management of money—other than salaries and grants—had small importance. The upheavals taking place in medicine today may cause faculties to change their values, but I doubt that this will happen. Because tradition—especially tradition that comes from a long line of able leaders—dies hard.

# 8
# On Being a Leader-Manager

Becoming leader-managers affected clinical chairs in many ways. It changed, for instance, their relation to the members of their departments. When the faculty at Stony Brook organized a faculty senate, members of our department understandably deemed me ineligible. I was management, they said, not faculty. "I fear," Giamatti wrote, "we will come to the point where the corporate structure will take over, where presidents, deans, chancellors, and lawyers will be constantly negotiating with the court on the one hand and with the faculty on the other" (43–44).

The move toward corporate structure also forced chairs to wrestle with an assortment of new questions. If, for example, faculty members fudged their costs of practice, should this be taken into account when the members came up for academic promotion? Should a reluctance to see indigent patients, patients who were a liability to the practice plan, be condemned or applauded?

I cannot speak for other chairs, but my attempts to both lead and manage produced schizophrenia: As a leader, I considered members of the department friends and colleagues; as a manager, money earners. As a leader, I expected members to teach, do research, and take care of patients, while as a manager I needed them to do procedures and fill beds. As a leader, I valued members for the ideas they generated; as a manager, for the dollars they brought in. And as a leader, I classified divisions according to their strength in teaching, research, and clinical care, but as a manager, I classified them as high or low earners.

Such schizophrenia, difficult for any leader to handle, would be especially difficult for clinical chairs. Their priceless heritage, handed down by chairs who led departments in the past, centered on scholarship, not business acumen. The William Oslers, Harvey Cushings, and Dickinson Richardses were known for being able to connect the narrow field of medicine to the great world of intellect and learning. Osler was at home in history and literature, Cushing won a Pulitzer Prize for biography, Richards wrote Latin and Greek.

Perhaps *scholar* is not quite the word to describe men and women like these. Perhaps we should instead say *civilized*, if we use the word in the way Edith Hamilton used it in *The Greek Way*. "Civilization," Hamilton wrote, "stands for a high matter quite apart from telephones and electric lights. It is a matter of imponderables, of delight in the things of the mind, of love of beauty, of honor, grace, courtesy" (1942, 106).

Present-day clinical chairs have little time for imponderables. They must instead be practical men and women who, as academic leaders, supervise teaching, patient care, and research. Then as managers they must maximize income, minimize expenses, ride herd on the costs of practice, and see that flows of patients are maintained. The number and diversity of these tasks make setting priorities difficult. It is hard to know which tasks should go at the top of the list.

The most successful chairs I've known have put people at the top. They've taken time to listen—really listen—to their students, interns, residents, fellows, and department members. They've pushed to get their young colleagues to the places they wanted to go. The chairs have done well, it seems to me, because they've seen to it that their departments more closely resembled families than businesses.

The successful chairs have, at the same time, maintained a realistic estimate of their own importance. In ordinary times, having a chair around is convenient but unnecessary. A department operates perfectly well when its chair is out of town. Chairs become useful when trouble starts—when, for instance, the president of the university gets fired, or the head of the hospital decides to move the cath labs from Medicine to Radiology. And a chair is especially useful if he or she has a knack for sensing trouble before it erupts. "When the evils that arise . . . are seen far ahead," wrote Machiavelli, "they are easily [cured]; but when [they] are allowed to grow [so] that they become manifest to every one, then they can no longer be remedied" (9).

And while helping people and handling crises, the successful chairs have kept the conversation going, the great conversation about goals, science, medicine, ideas—the civil conversation that is "tough, open, principled—between and among all members and parts of the institution." If the conversation is maintained, "a community is patiently built. If it is not, the place degenerates into a center of crisis management and competing special interests. What must be open and free is the conversation, between young and young, young and old, scholar and scholar, present and past—the sound of voices straining out the truth" (Giamatti, 45).

There is, incidentally, a redeeming feature of the myriad tasks a modern-day clinical chair must handle. The feature hinges on Karl Popper's view of the world, or, rather, his view that there are three worlds. Popper said that we spend our lives moving back and forth among the three—a world of objects, a world of sensations and emotions, and a world of products of the mind (1973, 54).

Chairs live with objects—needles, scalpels, stethoscopes. They stay immersed in emotions—a patient's pain, a family's anguish. And they continually deal with products of the mind—pressures, millimoles, balance sheets. Few jobs offer such variety. None brings more rewards.

# 9

# How Clinical Departments Acquired Six Conflicting Goals

Just as a new clinical chair inherits a tradition of scholarship, he or she also inherits six goals, things department members feel impelled to work toward. Some of the goals originated inside departments, while others came as responses to outside pressures, pressures departments were powerless to control. And, as might be expected of goals from different sources, some were in conflict with others, creating uncertainty in faculty members and giving chairs headaches.

I'll talk first about the origin of the goals, then about the uncertainty and headaches the goals continue to generate.

The opening of the Johns Hopkins Hospital and School of Medicine in the 1890s sparked a revolution in medical education in this country (Bordley and Harvey 1976, 132–34). The programs put in place by people like Osler, Halstead, Kelly, and Welch were innovative in the best sense of the word. Osler, for instance, said that senior medical students would serve as clinical clerks, and help take care of patients. The department would also offer postgraduate training to house physicians, the forerunners of the interns and residents we have today. Also, medicine would be taught at the bedside, through direct contact with patients, a startling change from the amphitheater demonstrations that had served as the backbone of teaching in the past.

The difference between Johns Hopkins and other schools was highlighted in 1910 when the Carnegie Foundation issued the *Flexner Report*. Of the 155 schools Flexner reviewed, Johns Hopkins alone required a candidate to have "a college degree which, whatever else it represents, must include the three fundamental sciences, French and German." After Johns Hopkins came fifteen schools that required at least two years of college. Then there were "about fifty schools" that asked for a high school education or its equivalent. The remaining schools asked "little or nothing more than the rudiments or the recollection of a common school education" (1972, 28–37). The Baltimore Medical College, for instance, required "much less than a four-year high school education" and often conferred advanced standing on students who flunked out of other schools (236).

The *Flexner Report* had a seismic effect on medical education. Standards were set and afterward enforced. Medical school departments became more like those at Johns Hopkins. And it is, I think, fair to say that Johns Hopkins, at the beginning of the century, gave clinical departments their two basic goals: to teach clinical medicine well, especially at the bedside, and to deliver the best possible patient care.

Research, at the time, was being carried out in clinical departments at Johns Hopkins and in the laboratories and hospital of the Rockefeller Institute. But these places were exceptions. The real flowering of research, the flowering that would make research a goal in clinical departments everywhere, still lay in the future.

In the 1920s and 1930s, sixty or so years after Claude Bernard had proclaimed that medicine was at last turning toward its permanent scientific path, there was little evidence that science had had much effect on the day-to-day practice of medicine. Physicians were using the fruits of clinical research—insulin and liver extract, for example—to treat their patients; but they were not yet relying much on measurements, other than for simple things like blood pressure, temperature, and blood cells. Reflecting in 1964, Dana Atchley provided insight into the state of things with his story of an incident at the College of Physicians and Surgeons in 1936:

> We were trying to teach the mechanisms of disease . . . rather than classify [each] with one word. But we were criticized. I'll never forget when I asked about the chloride content of the blood in an obscure case. One of our most brilliant men burst out and said, "You're just interested in a lot of laboratory data. You don't really care about the patient at all!" Which of course was not so, because we had always felt the patient was important. (108)

Science had not yet gained a foothold at the bedside.

But from the mid-1940s onward, things changed. For it was then that the National Institutes of Health began to pour into medical research and training the vast sums of money already mentioned. With this new emphasis on science, physicians were soon able to do such things as put numbers on renal function, evaluate the way the lungs and chest wall work, and measure pressures and rates of blood-flow through the heart and vessels. Everyday medicine, as Bernard had predicted, was becoming more quantitative.

And there would soon be sulfa, penicillin, oral diuretics, antitumor compounds, and antihypertensive agents. There would also be streptomycin, a drug that would help control tuberculosis, a scourge for five thousand years.

So under the stimulus of the National Institutes of Health, with its emphasis on science, members of clinical departments acquired their next two goals: to do research and to teach young people to do research.

The fifth goal came in the 1960s and was not directly connected to medicine. It was instead a product of politics, society, and the Vietnam War. As mentioned in section 5, the 1960s saw college students countrywide rebel against universities, government, and authority in general. The behavior of the students was so foreign to anything their elders had seen that it was hard for the elders to listen to the students, much less understand what the students were trying to say. It was especially hard for them to believe that the Vietnam War might be wicked, that the CIA might be doing things Americans criticized other governments for doing, and that the FBI was coming perilously close to violating the constitutional rights of people in this country. At the same time, people were being buffeted by two other crusades, both laudatory but unsettling. One was civil rights, the other feminism.

But how did these movements, especially the rebellion of the students, come to affect clinical departments? By causing young people to be introspective, to spend more time thinking about values and life-styles and personal goals than young men and women had ever done before. And the young people interested in medicine decided they would no longer work as interns, residents, or fellows for nominal salaries, as had been the custom in the past. Low salaries, they argued, placed an unfair burden on husbands, wives, and children. Similarly, the young people entering academic medicine wanted full-time salaries raised, then kept that way. These arguments were reinforced by the inflation of the 1960s and 1970s, a development that further reduced the value of take-home dollars. In responding to these outside pressures, schools and departments picked up a fifth goal: to raise full-time salaries and keep them high.

When clinical departments embraced goal 5, they automatically embraced a sixth goal, for in those days, the only way a department could keep salaries high, above the level covered by the university and by grants, was to do procedures and fill hospital beds. This was true because third-party carriers paid more for procedures and filled beds than for ambulatory care. So the last goal, a response to an outside pressure just as goal 5 had been, was to do procedures and fill beds.

The six goals, when pulled together, look like this:

1. To teach clinical medicine well, especially at the bedside.
2. To deliver the best possible patient care.
3. To do research.
4. To teach young people to do research.
5. To keep full-time salaries high.
6. To do procedures and fill beds.

With the exception of high salaries and the means of underwriting them, the goals were not new. They were much the same as the goals of clinical departments a half-century earlier. What was new was the way faculty members viewed the goals, the way they held all six to be equally important and refused to abandon any of them.

They did this even though some of the goals were in conflict with others. Faculty members found it hard, for instance, to fill beds and do procedures then have time left to do research and teach others to do it. There weren't enough hours for everything. So faculty members become uncertain about how to split their time. They wanted high salaries and were willing to earn them by seeing patients, but they knew that the safest way to promotion and tenure was by doing research.

The necessity of doing procedures and filling beds gave chairs headaches, for as we shall see in section 14, it placed an unfortunate emphasis on money and salaries, with the result that research and teaching could suffer.

There was, however, a feature of the goals that helped make the uncertainty and headaches bearable: clinical departments became more nearly balanced than ever before. In the early part of this century, clinicians held the upper hand; in the middle part, investigators did so. But in the 1970s and 1980s, when the six goals were all in place, a lucky chair had top-notch, full-time clinicians working alongside top-notch, full-time investigators, with each group aware of its dependence on the other.

Then came managed care. It has already tipped the balance sharply toward clinical practice and away from clinical research. And there is not, at the moment, any way to predict how far the tilt will go (section 41).

Before ending the discussion of goals, let's look for a moment at another term, *mission*. I have defined a *goal* as something department members feel impelled to work toward. Let's define *mission* as the reason for a department's existence, what a department is supposed to do.

Louis Welt, chair of medicine at the University of North Carolina, when chairing a meeting I attended in Washington in the 1970s, was asked, "What, exactly, do departments of medicine do?" After a few moments of thought, moments spent looking at the ceiling, Dr. Welt, speaking slowly, said, "They produce new knowledge, . . . they teach young people to produce more new knowledge, . . . and they teach other young people to apply the knowledge, both new and old."

Lou's words, sublime in their simplicity, defined the mission of all clinical departments, not just the mission of departments of medicine.

# 10
# Projects

Every chair will, from time to time, want to add goals to the six he or she inherited. But these new ventures, more often than not, will differ from the inherited goals in that the ventures will have a finite life span, usually weeks or months. I shall use the word *project* to describe goals that go out of existence when the tasks needed to accomplish them have been completed. A simple example would be persuading the dean to buy a heart-sound simulator for the faculty to use in teaching students. Once the dean has agreed to spend the money and the simulator has been purchased, the project ends. A more substantial project would be recruiting a division chief. When a candidate has been wooed, persuaded, and installed in office, the goal has been met.

Projects deserve our attention because they have importance over and above the improvements they produce. Properly designed and implemented, projects recreate the air of change and excitement that permeates departments when they are new. And big projects, like building a clinical research center, applying for a large training grant, or establishing a neighborhood outreach clinic, impart an aura of progress, of forward motion and growth.

Do all chairs need projects? Yes. Even chairs of departments that are eminently successful, because, as Peter Drucker tells us, non-profit organizations must—if they are to remain viable—either grow or find a substitute for growth. "Sooner or later," Drucker writes, "growth slows down and the institution plateaus. Then it has to be able to maintain its momentum, its flexibility, its vitality, and its vision" (1990, 10). Projects can do this.

## What Makes Projects Successful?

In thinking about projects, it's useful to keep in mind the way the educational piece of a clinical department differs from the business part. A business, Drucker says, supplies goods or services. It has accomplished its purpose when the customer buys its product and is satisfied with it. In contrast, a nonprofit agency supplies neither goods nor services. "Its 'product' is *a changed human being* . . . a child that learns, a young man or woman grown into a self-respecting adult" (xiv).

Projects in clinical departments need not always provide such lofty results, but they should, in one way or another, improve the lives or learning of students, house officers, faculty members, patients, or members of the administrative and technical staffs. A heart sound simulator could, as mentioned, do this, as could a new chief, the addition of a research center, or acquisition of a training grant.

I knew these things in a vague sort of way when I arrived at Stony Brook. And soon after my arrival, I decided that our first project would be to offer continuing medical education (CME) to the community hospitals on Long Island. We would send our specialists to the hospitals, and the specialists, in meetings like grand rounds, would bring the staff physicians at the hospitals up to date.

CME was, it seemed to me, the best possible project to start with, because it fitted the grand plan for our Health Sciences Center. The center was meant, the grand plan stipulated, to serve as a resource for all the patients, physicians, and hospitals on Long Island. Our project would also introduce our newly recruited physicians to their colleagues in the community.

It was a perfect project. So I launched it. And it failed. Miserably.

The failure might have been avoided if I had read Drucker before starting. Projects are, in essence, miniature goals or missions, and Drucker says a mission will fail—will fail without question—if you don't have three things: opportunities, competence, and commitment (8).

Did we have opportunities? Yes, I was sure of it. In those days, when CME was commanding nationwide attention, every community hospital wanted to mount the strongest educational program possible. But what I didn't know, because I hadn't bothered to ask, was that these hospitals, fiercely proud of their independence, wanted to design their own programs, not import programs from us. The opportunities I knew existed weren't there.

How about competence? Our specialists had competence. Lots of it.

And what about commitment? There was, as things turned out, none. Instead of talking the project through with members of the department, as I tried to do with most things, I had simply assumed that everyone would be interested in delivering CME. They would have to be, I reasoned, since CME in those days was touted as the future of American medicine. It would, experts assured us, keep physicians up to date, keep patients happy with their doctors, and convince the government that it need not bother to impose additional controls on the medical profession.

But I failed to recognize the obvious, namely, that newly recruited people in a young department have their hours filled with setting up labs, applying for grants, and all the other things involved in getting started. CME wasn't a top priority. It wasn't, in fact, a priority at all.

Our project had only one of the three essentials. So it was, as Drucker would have predicted, doomed.

Despite this first disaster, I soon learned the truth of something experts on management tell us: a well-run organization is goal and project directed, with people at the top who take pains to tell everyone what the goals and projects are. This approach keeps an organization focused on its mission. It prevents an organization from simply reacting to the daily crises that threaten to engulf it.

## The Role of Decision Making

Even when a leader who is considering a project holds planning sessions or consults widely with members of the organization, it is, in the end, the leader, and the leader alone, who decides whether a project should be launched. "It's in the decision," Drucker wrote, "that everything comes together. That is the make or break point of the organization. Most of the other tasks executives do, other people can do. But only executives can make the decisions" (121). Pierre Mendes-France drove the point home in a single terse statement: "To govern is to choose" (Schlesinger 1993, 39).

A clinical chair decides not only which projects to start but also which ones to abandon, either because the projects aren't working or because they are no longer useful. Abandoning a project is harder than starting one, because it forces a leader to choose between the embarrassment of admitting failure and the cost of further loss of time and effort. Abandonment is especially hard for clinical chairs,

because people in nonprofit organizations tend to consider everything they do to be righteous and moral (Drucker 1990, 10–11).
Hence, abandoning a project is, for a clinical chair, like violating a
trust.

## Attitudes toward Change

A successful project will change something, and all of us, to some
extent, are wary of change of any sort. Eric Hoffer tells a story about
our fear of change: Back in 1936, he spent a good part of the year
picking peas. He started in early January, in the Imperial Valley, and
later drifted northward as the fields of peas ripened. Then in June,
when the peas were gone, he started to pick string beans. "And I still
remember," Hoffer said, "how hesitant I was that first morning as I
was about to address myself to the string bean vines. Would I be able
to pick string beans? Even the change from peas to string beans had
in it elements of fear" (1963, 1).

Most clinical chairs would, I suspect, sympathize with Hoffer. For
clinical chairs are known for their devotion to standing pat. In his
1962 presidential address at the Association of American Physicians,
Dickinson W. Richards, Jr., quoting an earlier president of the association, issued the ringing, tongue-in-cheek declaration, "The major
purpose of the Association of American Physicians is to resist
change" (1). Along these same lines, Clark Kerr is said to have remarked that trying to change a university curriculum is like trying
to move a cemetery.

A department's attitude toward change depends in part on the
department's age. I learned this when I decided to leave P and S and
go to Stony Brook. For six months after making the decision, I spent
mornings in the city at P and S and afternoons on Long Island at
Stony Brook. The contrast was startling. Each morning I would try
to shove the small part of P and S where I had influence one millime-
ter off the course it had been on for many years and intended to
stay on for many more. Each afternoon I would try to apply enough

restraints at Stony Brook to keep our new department from flying apart. The contrast between the old and the new made me notice the different attitudes toward change. People at P and S were wary of change, as people at established schools tend to be. People at Stony Brook regarded change as a way of life.

But why should making changes be more difficult in older schools? I decided—rightly or wrongly—that the answer lay in the fear of damaging tradition, of altering things put in place by the giants of the past. And if, by chance, a change was made, it immediately became part of the tradition, so even if the change made things worse, not better, there was a reluctance to go back to the way things were. The medical school at Stony Brook had two things going for it: there weren't any giants to worry about, and tradition didn't exist.

But back to projects. Machiavelli tells us that Ferdinand of Aragon "was always planning great enterprises, which kept the minds of his subjects in a state of suspense and admiration, and occupied with their results. And these different enterprises followed so quickly one upon the other, that he never gave [the people] a chance deliberately to make any attempt against himself" (98–99). Ferdinand understood the importance of projects. He knew they enhanced the well-being of his people and ensured his own personal safety, two items that are, for any leader, primal concerns.

# *11*
# Departments as Loosely
# ˌ Coupled Systems

A clinical department that has divisions or sections usually operates as a loosely coupled system (LCS), a type of organization that has been described in several ways (Orton and Weick, 1990). Glassman (1973), for instance, said that loose coupling exists if the elements of a system have few variables in common or if the common variables are weak compared to other variables that influence the system. Weick (1976) wrote that with loose coupling the elements of a system are responsive to each other but retain evidence of separateness and identity. Weick later (1982) expanded his definition by detailing the ways that loosely coupled elements can interact.

For the purposes of this section I define loose coupling as existing when the elements of a system operate with considerable autonomy and an event in one element can affect any or all of the others. Analyzing a clinical department with these features in mind sheds light on the job of a clinical chair.

Take, for instance, a chair and his or her home department (a system), made up of chiefs and their divisions (the system's elements). Each division will have its own research interests, its own grants, and its own ancillary personnel. The chair will reign over a federation of divisions, of semi-independent strongholds, rather than a single unified group. Hence, the chair is in a position quite different from that of, say, the CEO of a traditional, profit-making enterprise. Such a CEO, Larry Hirschhorn points out, usually has enough control of resources and personnel to enable him or her to plan the course the enterprise will be taking. A clinical chair, in contrast, can lay plans, but the plans will usually be aimed at "protecting and guiding the system," rather than detailing its future course (1995, 2).

To protect the system, the leader has to manage the contradictions that exist in the LCS and handle the conflicts that arise among its parts. The leader tries to hold the parts together, to keep the whole intact. So leaders don't really direct the system so much as they "insure that it remains upright" (2).

The leader protects the system in another way: if a crisis develops in one part, the leader tries to keep the crisis localized, to keep the trouble from infecting other units, to hold "the system within its safety zone." One way to do this, suggested Hirschhorn, is to jot down a series of scenarios, each describing a way the system might be pushed beyond its limits. The collection then becomes the basis for planning, problem solving, and crisis management (2).

Guiding an LCS, the second duty of the leader, cannot be done by using "the familiar tools of controlling and allocating the systems' capital, expenses or investments" (3). The leader has to guide the system in more subtle ways. A wise chair does this, more often than not, by first looking for consensus, and by then nudging the consensus in the direction the chair wants it to go.

Hirschhorn recommended that a steering committee be used to help guide the system, and I can, from my experience at Stony Brook, endorse this idea (see section 12). He suggested a small committee, say, a half-dozen members; but in a department with ten or more divisions, the committee has to be larger, to insure that all the subunits have a voice. Also, the projects planned by the committee should be of interest to as many subunits as possible.

Finally, the leader can guide the system by "operating at the seams," at the edges of the various units, in regions that are not claimed by anyone (4). A chair can, for example, arrange seminars, with speakers whose work would be of interest to more than one unit. The chair can also promote such things as departmentwide research conferences.

Whether or not a chair's home department has divisions or sections, the chair may be the leader of another LCS, comprising the chairs and their departments at affiliated hospitals. These combinations would, I think, usually qualify as LCSs, and the points already mentioned about an LCS made up of divisions would also apply to an LCS made up of affiliated departments.

The very nature of loosely coupled systems is one of contradiction and conflict, a statement borne out by two decades worth of books and articles on LCSs, mostly on those found in education. The statement is also borne out by years of experience in clinical departments. The origins of conflict in departments include, the tension between divisions that feature research and those that feature clinical care, and between divisions that are handsomely reimbursed, for doing procedures, and those that are short-changed, because they rely on cognitive skills.

There is no question that conflict can, at times, be a good thing. I mentioned, in section 4, that debates, complaints, and arguments keep the department's pot of energy boiling; and in section 5 I quoted Thomas Jefferson's assertion that conflict is necessary if a democratic government is to stay strong. At a less important level, conflict can help a chair take the measure of the members of his or her department. Watching a member argue an issue in public is a fine way to gauge the member's maturity: Are the comments balanced? thought through? logical? So, while the members debate and argue, the chair makes mental notes on their strengths, weaknesses, and vulnerabilities.

But where should a chair draw the line between good conflict and bad? The line is crossed, a friend suggested, whenever conflict triggers talk or action that damages another person or threatens the welfare of the group. Members of the French National Assembly of 1789 would have approved of my friend's view. When the authors drafted the Declaration of the Rights and Duties of Man and Citizens, they included the line, "Liberty consists of being able to do whatever is not injurious to the rights of others."

What should a chair do when conflict upsets a department member so much that he or she goes around the chair to the dean? A fellow chair told me that when this happens, she calls the guilty person in and says, "From now on, the matter's between you and the dean. No need for me to waste my time on something you two are handling."

There is a vast literature on dealing with conflict, because conflict has, for many years, been a popular topic with psychologists, psychiatrists, and experts on management. Tucker, in his book *Chairing the Academic Department* (1992), has a long chapter on conflict, with a bibliography of forty books and articles. So anyone wishing to read a detailed discussion of conflict in academic circles may want to consult Tucker's book.

There is, though, one technique for handling conflict that I want to mention, a technique described by Peter Drucker, who cites the work of Mary Parker Follet, a psychologist who lived in the early part of this century. Ms. Follet said that when arguments arise, a leader should never ask who is right or what is right. Instead, the leader should assume that each party is giving a right answer but to a different question. Then, if the leader can figure out the questions, the leader may be able to tone down the argument (1990, 124).

Robert McAfee Brown (1955) used this approach when discussing the celebrated argument about the origin of the universe. "Who is right," Brown asked, "the 'religionists' or the 'scientists'? To ask the question this way (as we usually do) is to miss the point." The religionists "are dealing with the religious question, 'Why?' Why the world?" The answer, Brown says, is, "Because God in his greatness and love has brought it into being." The evolutionists, on the other hand, are dealing with the question, "How?" And here, Brown says, we must turn to scientists for answers (1955, 60).

It's always a good idea to give Follet's approach a try, for even when the approach fails to settle the argument, it helps to clarify the opposing views.

When, in the middle years of this century, many clinical departments abandoned the idea of an absolute chair and installed a chair with chiefs, the departments moved from tight to loose coupling, and in doing this, moved toward contradictions and conflict. Even so, loose coupling has served departments well. It has given members a fine blend of constraint and independence and has proved to be adaptable to diverse styles of leadership, ranging from relaxed permissiveness to rigid control.

## 12
## Committees and Democracy

Members of democratic societies pride themselves on being individualists. Yet, democracies are, to a considerable extent, run by groups. The Senate, Supreme Court, and House of Representatives play essential roles in our federal government. And in present-day clinical departments, committees carry out assignments that would be hard to handle in any other way.

I shall begin by describing the committees that exist in a typical home department. Most of what I say will also apply to committees in affiliated departments, though, of course, no two departments—home or affiliated—will be structured in exactly the same way.

## Types of Committees

### *The Advisory Committee*

Every clinical chair, at one time or another, has turned to friends or colleagues for help and advice. The practice of using a handful of senior faculty members as informal consultants (see section 2), was, I am told, widespread during the middle part of this century. But by the late 1950s and early 1960s, clinical departments had entered the era of explosive growth mentioned earlier; and as this growth continued, chairs began putting together organized groups to advise them in more formal ways.

The group in our home department at Stony Brook—a group called the advisory committee (AC)—was similar, I later learned, to those in home departments chaired by others I knew. The members of our AC included the chair and vice chair, the ten division chiefs, the supervisor of the clerkship, the supervisor of the residency program, our representative to the practice plan, and the head of the clinical practice committee. In addition to these sixteen people—all members of the AC because of the positions they held in the department—there were three elected members, who served staggered, two-year terms.

As things turned out, having elected members on the committee was a good idea. The turnover they provided helped prevent the committee from becoming fossilized. And though the chiefs were supposed to relay the deliberations of the committee to the rest of the faculty, the elected members did a better job of this. I also had the impression that the faculty preferred to talk to the elected members when they had issues they wanted brought to the committee's attention.

The AC met once a month, with an agenda sent to each member in advance of the meeting. The topics, as characterized by one of the members at the time, were "the things at the home base the chair can't handle by himself." Hence, the topics included faculty recruitment, projects, allocation of practice income, the status of research, and the cause and elimination of trouble spots. The discussions were spirited and free-wheeling. At many meetings, the air was thick with ideas, proposals, and counterproposals.

Were any members of the AC unhappy with the committee? Yes. On one occasion or another, a member would complain that the executive committee of the department was handling issues that rightly belonged in the AC. The complaints were always valid or partly valid, because the issues the two committees dealt with were closely related. The difference was that the AC dealt with activities at the home base, while the executive committee—with representatives from the affiliates as well as from the home base (see section 6)—dealt with issues of departmentwide importance. Hence, the executive committee handled things like appointments and promotions, assignment of students to the different hospitals, and (in the interest of uniformity) evaluation of clerks and subinterns at the various training sites. Occasionally, a member of the AC would grumble about some other inadequacy of the committee, but by and large, the committee worked well.

### The Departmental Tenure Committee

Unlike the AC, which had multiple duties, our tenure committee did just one thing: it decided who, in our department, should be nominated for tenure. The final decision about tenure came, of course, from the trustees of the university, on the advice of a universitywide tenure committee, but our departmental committee served as a useful first step in selecting the candidates whose names would be sent forward.

Our committee consisted of all the tenured people in the department, a number that, at the time I was chair, was sixteen. That we had only sixteen tenured people was a stroke of fortune, because a larger committee might not have worked so well. We agreed that the members of the committee would elect one of their number to preside, and we also agreed that I would attend meetings as an ex officio member.

We operated along the same lines as the school's tenure committee. We appointed a three-person ad hoc committee to gather information on each person being considered. Members of the ad hoc committee solicited letters and sought opinions of the candidate from tenured people, both inside and outside our school. And if the ad hoc committee gave a favorable report and the discussion of the report by the entire tenure committee was also favorable, I forwarded our recommendation to the dean.

Not all clinical departments have tenure committees. One reason, I suspect, is the uneven distribution of tenured people among divisions or units. This can present a problem, because people in divisions and groups have a habit of voting as a bloc. They are more likely to do this if the candidate comes from a rival division, a rivalry based, say, on who will take care of patients with lymphoma. But so long as each tenured member votes his or her personal opinion, the system works.

In section 35 I mention my uncertainty about whether tenure should be continued. But if a school does continue it, the most capable people on the faculty should help choose the candidates, for the future of a department, school, or university depends directly on the quality of its permanent faculty.

## The Clinical Practice Committee

There are many types of clinical practice committees, some focused on in-patient services, some on ambulatory medicine, some on the income from patient care, and some on other aspects of a faculty's clinical practice. But there is one type of practice committee that should be in every department: a committee that brings nurses and physicians together, on a regular basis, to discuss how the delivery of care is going. The committee may also include pharmacists, social workers, community practitioners, hospital administrators, and representatives of other disciplines. But whatever the composition, the committee must provide an opportunity for nurses and physicians, at the very least, to discuss the care of patients once or twice a month.

The responsibilities of such a committee are so obvious that it isn't necessary to list them. Besides, the committee's most important purpose would not appear on the list. That purpose is to keep doctors and nurses in contact, to keep them sharing problems, to keep them talking to each other.

## Residency and Clerkship Committees

Every department with interns and residents will have a residency committee, headed by the chair or someone the chair designates. The make-up of the committee will depend on the requirements of the licensing board of the particular specialty, and so, to a considerable extent, will the committee's duties. But despite differences in membership and duties, every such committee will have evaluating the performance of interns and residents as its chief responsibility. The committee may also arrange remedial help, plan changes in the training schedule, and advise the chair, at the end of the year, about who should be promoted to the next level of training. The committee may also help the chair decide which of the residents completing their training should write the certifying examination.

Departments that offer clerkships for students may or may not have a clerkship committee. If there is one, the members will do much the same things as the people on residency committees—evaluate performance, arrange remedial help, and the like. If the department does not have a formal committee, the director of the clerkship, in putting together evaluations, will enlist the aid of attendings who have made rounds with the students.

When thinking about our experience with clerks at Stony Brook, my memory often flips back to an afternoon when Martin Liebowitz, director of our clerkship program and vice chair of the department of medicine, met with a small group of clerks to hear one of them, a young man, present a patient. When the young man finished, Marty asked:

"In the light of what you've found, Erik, do you think the diagnosis should be changed?"

"No."

"Should we, Erik, add other drugs?"

"No."

"Well then, Erik, is there anything at all you want to tell us?"

"Yes. My name's not Erik."

## Two Problems and a Suggestion

Everything I've said to this point has underscored the importance of committees in clinical departments. Yet, committees—both inside and outside of medical schools—have serious flaws. Anyone who has served on a committee will know about these weaknesses and will also know that two of the main problems are the behavior of individual people and the way people relate to each other when working as a group.

Lewis Thomas, with his usual insight, wrote about the first flaw, the behavior of individual people. In his book, *The Medusa and the Snail*, Thomas pointed out that at the start of a committee meeting

> each person is necessarily an actor, uncontrollably acting out the part of himself, reading the lines that identify him, asserting his identity. This takes quite a lot of time, and while it is going on, there is little chance of anything else getting done. . . . We are designed, coded, it seems, to place the highest priority on being individuals, and we must do this first, at whatever cost, even if it means disability for the group. (1979, 155–16)

A chair can sometimes thwart this individualistic behavior by first calling the meeting to order and then immediately writing on the blackboard the first item of business to be considered. After this, the chair can, with tact and diplomacy, ask people who begin to act out their personalities how their comments bear on the written target.

Irving Janis wrote about the second flaw, the trouble that can grow out of relationships between people. In his book *Victims of Groupthink*, Janis said:

> In my . . . research on group dynamics, I was impressed by repeated manifestations of the effects—both favorable and unfavorable—of the social pressures that typically develop in cohesive groups—in infantry platoons, air crews, therapy groups, seminars, and self-study or encounter groups of executives receiving leadership training. In all these groups . . . members tend to evolve informal objectives to preserve friendly intragroup relations and this becomes a part of the hidden agenda of their meetings. (1972, 8)

This second flaw, the development of bonds between committee members, can be controlled in part by changing the committee's membership from time to time, as we did with the elected members in our AC. The effect of the flaw can also be reduced, suggested Janis, by having a parallel group consider the same topics (211). We did this by means of a junior advisory committee, a group I shall describe when we talk about faculty (section 33).

The two flaws just mentioned grow out of the act of coming together, of committee members meeting as a group. To eliminate the necessity of holding meetings, Lewis Thomas suggested using the Delphi technique, in which the leader, instead of calling meetings, sends a questionnaire to each member, and the member writes out answers and sends the questionnaire back. After collating the answers, the leader sends a copy to each member, and the member, after thinking over the answers the others have given, fills out the questionnaire again. Then the process is repeated until some sort of consensus forms. In Thomas's experience, three cycles are usually enough.

The Delphi technique, wrote Thomas,

> is a really quiet, thoughtful conversation in which everyone gets a chance to *listen*. The background noise of small talk, and the recurrent sonic booms of vanity, are eliminated at the outset, and there is time to think. There are no voices, and therefore no rising voices. It is, when you look at it in this way, a great discovery. Before Delphi, real listening in a committee meeting had always been a near impossibility. Each member's function was to talk, and while other people were talking the individual member was busy figuring out what he ought to say next in order to shore up his own original position. Debating is what committees really do, not thinking. Take away the need for winning points, leading the discussion, protecting one's face, gaining applause, shouting down opposition, scaring opponents, all that kind of noisy activity, and a group of bright people can get down to quiet thought. It is a nice idea, and I'm glad it works. (188–19)

## Decision Making

There is another problem with committees, a problem different from the flaws I've mentioned, and it is that discussions in committees, or in group meetings of any sort, seldom end in unanimity. This means that the chair has to extract from the various opinions a single policy or decision, and the obvious way to do this is to call for a vote.

When anyone mentions voting, I think back to a conversation that took place about twenty years ago, shortly after I had been appointed chair. At a cocktail party in Washington, I talked about decision making with two old friends, Joe Reeves, then chair of medicine at Alabama, and Helen Ranney, then chair of medicine at La Jolla. "I've learned," I said, "to be content with 51 percent of the vote." "In a department of medicine," Joe declared, "51 percent is both a plurality and a majority!" "Why would you let them vote?" Helen asked.

Later, when I had had more experience, I discovered that Helen's question—asked in jest—was the wisest possible course. Votes can be deadly traps that commit chairs to policies they had no intention of adopting. If a chair has any hope of controlling democracy, he or she will never call for a vote unless the issue is trivial, and will head off votes proposed by others unless absolutely certain the votes will come out the way the chair wants them to. Deciding an issue by discussion, and then consensus, is a far safer way to set policy and make decisions.

Regardless of the efficiency of its committees and other such bodies, a democratic government won't work well without a strong leader. This fact has been known since antiquity and demonstrated repeatedly by our American presidents. Democratic governments, whether national or departmental, need strong leaders as badly as monarchies need them.

Jean Bodin (1958), the sixteenth-century French political theorist, believed that one political institution, be it king, leader, or legislative group, had to be endowed with ultimate authority if the government was to be strong. In a democratic clinical department, the chair must have this authority. While promoting the idea of democracy, the chair must keep the reins of power in his or her hands.

Do my suggestions for countering flaws and avoiding votes subvert the principles of democracy? Perhaps, but the suggestions may also subvert a greater evil, an evil that Friedrich Nietzsche mentioned (Janis, 3): madness, Nietzsche said, is rare in individuals but the rule in groups.

# 13
# Veterans Hospitals and Medical Schools

An affiliation between a Veterans Administration hospital and a medical school almost always benefits both parties. At the VA end, for instance, an affiliation makes it easier to recruit M.D.s and build a house officer program, while at the school end, an affiliation provides, among other things, additional faculty and a rich source of patients for teaching students, interns, and residents.

Our affiliation with the Northport VA hospital brought an even greater benefit: it enabled our department to survive. As mentioned earlier, our university hospital and health sciences center weren't completed for seven years after our department was organized; and during those years, the Northport VA served as our home. We recruited faculty, taught students, trained house officers, and got research projects going thanks to the VA's kindness in housing us. And when our university quarters were at last completed, many of the programs we put in place were extensions of programs we had started at the veterans hospital.

Once we had both the VA and university parts running, we wanted the two groups of people to be, as nearly as possible, one faculty. To this end, we used the same procedure for recruiting staff members at the two places and the same committee for reviewing candidates being considered for appointments or promotions. We alternated our weekly grand rounds between the two hospitals and brought the staffs together for death and discharge conferences once a month. And if the chief of a division received his or her salary from a VA line, then an associate chief was, in most instances, on a medical school line, and vice versa.

There was, however, one barrier to integration that we could neither eliminate nor minimize: half of our people received salaries from the VA and half received salaries from the medical school. This was a barrier because the salaries paid to junior people at the VA were higher than those paid junior people at the school, while the salaries paid to senior people differed in the other direction. These differences caused unhappiness, because, in promoting the idea of one faculty, we often had VA and medical school M.D.s working shoulder to shoulder but being paid at different rates. The salary barrier to integration was even worse for departments like surgery. Here, both junior and senior VA salaries were below those paid by medical schools across the country.

Another troublesome barrier was that a full-time Veterans Administration M.D. was not supposed to see nonveteran patients, except under special circumstances. This meant that those doctors were ineligible to join the school practice plan, a step that would, at least in theory, have enabled us to eliminate the differences in salaries. We talked about making those full-time M.D.s part-time, but the doctors themselves were against the change. Some of the reasons had to do with benefits and bonuses, but the chief reason was that if the VA Central Office decided to reduce the number of M.D.s in the VA system, as the Central Office had sometimes done, M.D.s on part-time lines were the first to go.

The dilemma I've just mentioned existed in other schools' affiliations with VA hospitals, not just ours. And no one has spoken to the dilemma—or to other features of affiliations—with more insight than Robert Petersdorf did in an article entitled "The VA–Medical School Partnership: The Medical School Perspective" (1987)*:

---

*Excerpts reprinted by permission of *American Medicine* (formerly *Journal of Medical Education*) and the Association of Medical Colleges.

I would like to suggest that all appointments of physicians at VA hospitals affiliated with medical schools be on a basis of no more than seven-eighths, whereby the physician is obligated to devote seven-eighths of the workweek to the VA and is free to work for the academic medical center. This will permit the VA to reduce its salaries and bonus payments accordingly and provide a better justification for the medical school and its practice plan to pay VA physicians. In many ways, this is much better than maintaining an arrangement whereby full-time VA physicians are paid supplements by the medical schools. Moreover, full-time arrangements lead to a degree of separatism between VA physicians and medical school faculty members that is neither necessary nor desirable. By having all faculty members work on a seven-eighths basis, they could legally be called upon to work on medical school matters off-site. . . . The medical school should also provide for differences in perquisites. . . . Likewise, the VA should be working toward a sabbatical leave policy similar to its parent medical school, and conversely the medical school should guarantee sabbaticals to VA-based faculty members. (154)

Had we had a plan like this, our problems would have been solved, for if all of our VA M.D.s had become part-time, as Dr. Petersdorf suggested, they could have joined our practice plan, and could also have quit worrying about being fired before full-timers, because there wouldn't have been any full-timers around. And now, several years after Dr. Petersdorf wrote his paper, many departments, as I understand it, have placed their VA M.D.s on part-time lines.

So much, for the moment, about the school end of affiliations. What do VA directors think about partnerships with schools? Mirvis et al. conducted a survey, published in 1994, in which they queried VA directors, associate directors, and chiefs of staff about their views on affiliation. Each person was asked whether he or she agreed or disagreed with each of the following statements:

1. Affiliations have a net positive effect to the VA.
2. Affiliates divert resources away from the major goals of the VA toward their own goals.

3. Affiliates help the VA recruit high quality physicians.
4. The VA should promote affiliations.
5. Faculty appointments for VA physicians reduce the effectiveness of VA physicians in meeting the goals of the VA.
6. The VA should prohibit salary supplementation of VA staff by universities.
7. VA staff physicians in affiliated hospitals are treated as "second-class citizens" by the university.
8. The VA should discourage new affiliations. (163)*

When the survey was completed, Mirvis and his colleagues analyzed the answers in several ways, but the results, viewed overall, showed "strongly positive general attitudes toward VA-university affiliations" by all three groups of administrators. At the same time, the results revealed concerns that affiliations were causing resources to be diverted from the VA and toward university goals and that VA-based faculty held a lower status.

Dr. Petersdorf mentions these points in one of the closing paragraphs of his paper, where he expressed the hope that VAs and their parent university hospitals will "do more to help one another." He pointed out that VA–medical school agreements "have often favored the parent hospital rather than the VA," and he suggested some remedies.

Where possible, a parent hospital should sign contracts with the VA on terms favorable to the VA and should not force the VA hospital to contract with nonaffiliated community hospitals. On the personnel side, I would hope for a closer working relationship between the directors and chiefs of staffs at VA hospitals and their counterparts in university teaching hospitals or other public hospitals affiliated with the university. To cement these relationships, I hope that schools will appoint their VA chiefs of staff as associate deans and have them function as integral members of the deanery. Likewise, I would like to

*Copyright Southern Society for Clinical Investigation, Inc., reprinted by permission of Lippincott-Raven Publishers.

see stronger administrative relationships forged between the hospital directors and the administration of academic medical centers. This means that the academic medical centers need to give their VA colleagues a bigger voice in medical school decision making, and I hope this will come to pass. (1987, 157)

In October 1996, the VA Central Office notified its hospitals that a new eligibility reform bill made it possible for full-time VA physicians to see private patients. Though it is too early to know how the bill will work, it should be a plus for affiliations.

Meanwhile, VAs and schools should use Dr. Petersdorf's paper as a guide for planning. The changes he suggests are what affiliations need. A few revisions in rules, plus a generous measure of goodwill, could make an enormous difference. And deans and directors, with a little effort, could make this difference real.

# 14
# Money

The worst effect of converting clinical departments to corporations was just what Giamatti said—a loss of collegiality. And nowhere did this loss produce more hard feelings than in the setting of salaries. In the academic world of the past, the world whose loss Giamatti lamented, salaries were tied to seniority and achievements, not earning power. But from the 1960s onward, earning power became an important factor; and thanks to the distorted scales of third-party carriers, the amount of money a department member could earn depended on the specialty or subspecialty the member was in. Those in fields with lots of procedures (e.g., surgery or medical cardiology) could bring in more dollars than people in disciplines with few procedures (e.g., psychiatry or endocrinology). According to the all-powerful third-party carriers, manual dexterity was worth top dollar but thinking only minimal scale.

The problem for clinical chairs was that extradepartmental agencies—third-party carriers—were dictating intradepartmental policy. Faculty members competed on equal terms in research and teaching and were rewarded according to standards set by the department, but when it came to doing procedures and filling beds, the carriers set the standards, and in doing this, made equally able physicians unequal.

To determine the range of earning power in our department of medicine, I stole an idea from Harold Fallon, chair of medicine at Virginia Commonwealth School of Medicine, and constructed a table. In the first column, I listed a dozen or so services our department offered, from working up an ambulatory patient, through procedures like gastroscopy, to procedures like coronary angiography. In a second column, I noted the amount of money our third-party carriers would pay for each service. Then in a third column I entered an estimate of the time required to perform the service for an average, uncomplicated patient. Finally, I divided the payment by the time required to perform the service and placed these calculated figures in column four.

The calculated numbers, the payment a staff member could earn per hour, stretched from $60 to $600. Needless to say, when the time came each spring to set salaries, the high earners argued fiercely that they deserved larger raises than those who earned less.

Still following Fallon's lead, I took data for the preceding fiscal year and tabulated the dollars each member of the department had earned. Then I divided the people into four groups: instructors, assistant professors, associate professors, and professors. And when I plotted the earnings according to rank, I found what Fallon had found—a striking inverse relationship. The lower the rank, the greater the amount of money he or she had brought in. The graphed points made it clear that it was junior faculty members who spent the most hours doing procedures and filling beds.

As a leader, I realized that these junior people were the ones who should be spending their time building reputations in research and teaching. But as a manager I knew that if the young people quit earning money, we would have to slash salaries across the board.

Our practice plan was new at the time and did not, as yet, contain provisions for setting salary supplements according to earnings. So, with the help and advice of the chiefs, I set the salaries for all of the members of the department, drawing from a pot of money the dean had given me for this purpose. As a rule of thumb, I kept the salaries of people with the same rank and similar accomplishments within 15 percent of each other, placing the high earners or grant winners at the top of the 15 percent range, the low earners at the bottom, and the rest in between. The narrow range evoked cries of anguish from the high earners, and I felt bad about that. But thinking back, I'm not sure the scheme was as unsatisfactory as the high earners believed it was.

Even after our practice plan had evolved into a system that connected earnings with salary supplements, I found it a good idea to look again, from time to time, at the graph that related earnings to academic rank. The graph was a painful reminder that our junior members were shouldering the biggest part of the clinical load. Chairs have always had to protect young faculty members from too many committees and too many other administrative tasks. And from the time the first practice plan went into operation, chairs have had to protect their young people from devoting too many hours to patient care.

## Personnel

When hard and soft dollars are added together, the total budget of a modern clinical department may exceed eight figures. Yet, these huge sums are often handled by administrative assistants, who get neither proper titles nor appropriate salaries. In 1975 Eugene Braunwald carried out a remarkably informative study in which he compared the salaries of financial personnel in clinical departments to the salaries of financial executives in businesses with comparable budgets and similar size. Dr. Braunwald found that the average salary of an administrative assistant in a clinical department was about 25 percent of the salary of the chair. In contrast, the average salary of a financial person in a business was 75 percent of the chief executive's salary.

Though Dr. Braunwald published his study twenty years ago, I doubt that things are much different in many places today. Salaries for financial executives in clinical departments have always been hard to come by. So keeping track of money can still be one of a chair's heaviest loads. But a wise chair, these days, will bring onto the staff someone trained in finance, to build, organize, and then watch over the business section of the department. Instead of calling the person an administrative assistant, as has been the custom in the past, the chair should give the person a title like vice chair for finance. And before recruiting this person, a chair may want to take a look at an article by J. S. Emrich entitled "Alternative Organizational Structures for a Department of Medicine" (1992). The article is a highly readable story about an imaginary clinical chair who realizes that his department needs restructuring and calls in an expert on management to advise him.

Even if a chair recruits an expert to handle finances, the chair will want to be able to read and understand the department's books. To this end, the chair might try *Finance and Accounting for Nonfinancial Managers*, by S. A. Finkler (1992), a small paperback that was used as a text at the 1995 AAMC Executive Development Seminar. Finkler defines financial terms so clearly that the book can, I believe, be read and understood by anyone, even those of us who are blissfully ignorant of the most fundamental principles of finance.

## Practice Plans

Since no two practice plans are the same, it would be foolish to offer a detailed discussion of the subject, even if I were competent to do this. Besides, plans are generally so complex that a small monograph would, I imagine, be required to cover all the parts of any one plan anywhere. But there are two features of practice plans that are, in my experience and in the experience of friends, worth considering for any plan.

One feature is that the money brought into the department through grants—or, at least, the part that helps pay salaries—should be credited to the person and the division who won it, in the same way that the money would be credited if it were earned by seeing patients. The other feature is the one already mentioned: there should be a recognizable relation between the money a person brings in and the person's take-home pay.

There is a third feature, a feature more controversial than the two just mentioned, that is an essential part of most practice plans. It has to do with ceilings and the tax on overage. A faculty member is usually given a ceiling on annual earnings. Any portion earned in excess of that amount is called overage, and it is customary to tax the overage in some way. The question is: should the rate of taxation rise or fall as the overage increases? If the tax increases as overage goes up (e.g., 10% on the first $500, 20% on the second, etc.), there will be little incentive to do extra work, because the extra dollars will, in increasing numbers, go to the school or to another person's salary. But these diminishing returns, some chairs like to believe, may persuade the person to forget about earning money and turn his or her attention to other things, like research. If, on the other hand, the rate of taxation falls as overage rises, there is incentive to do extra work, and thus bring money to the department.

Some schools favor one scheme, some the other. It's a hard decision but one that every school with ceilings and overage in its practice plan must make.

## Handling Practice Income

Chairs everywhere, I suspect, control expenditures of hard money, but the control of the soft money left over after salary supplements have been set and allocations put aside for running the department, varies from place to place and time to time. In a department that has division chiefs, a chair decides, at, say, the beginning of the fiscal year, who will hold the bulk of the remaining soft money—the chair or the chiefs.

A chair who opts to hold the money will retain an important measure of control but will, at the same time, be forced to listen to continual petitions for funds from the chiefs. A chair may, therefore, be willing to distribute the extra dollars among the divisions and let the chiefs control the money, in exchange for the tranquillity this move will buy.

During one week several years ago, a half-dozen desk-top computers were stolen from rooms in our department. The burglar had a master key. The security guards began searching for the burglar, then suggested that while the search was in progress, we should change all our locks. The department had almost a hundred rooms, with more than a hundred locks—all large, all expensive, and all costly to remove and replace. When our chiefs heard what the guards recommended, they sent memos to my office requesting that I underwrite changing every lock in the place. Thank goodness we had agreed earlier that they, the chiefs, would control most of the soft money. I could happily remind them that since they, not I, held the dollars, they could decide how much security they wanted to buy.

In addition to deciding who would hold the money, we had to decide how the practice income would be apportioned among high- and low-earning divisions. At the time I faced this issue, third party schedules of reimbursement were set so that two allergists who saw twenty ambulatory patients in a morning made less money than one cardiologist, working with one patient in the cardiac catheterization laboratory. To counter such an imbalance, we devised a formula for apportioning income that gave divisions credit for the number of patients seen, as well as for the amount of money earned. The formula helped, but the root problem remained. Even though reimbursement schedules have, in recent years, been more equitable, bothersome differences continue to exist.

### Funding Research

Since the late 1940s, members of clinical departments have, in a very real sense, been in partnership with the National Institutes of Health. The NIH, wanting to improve the health of the American people, has given clinical investigators huge sums of money to carry out the necessary research.

The investigators, although sharing the NIH's wish to improve health, have, at the same time, used research to build reputations and earn promotions. Hence, the partnership has been a happy, fruitful arrangement that has contributed, in a major way, to the extra twenty or so years of life expectancy that Americans have been given during this century.

In addition to obtaining funds from the NIH, clinical investigators have gotten money from other sources, like foundations, industries, government contracts, and partnerships with national laboratories. And now, with the worry that the trend toward smaller government will reduce the dollars available from the NIH, investigators are more than ever turning to these other sources for help (Eaton 1995).

Let's consider, for a moment, the difference between being in partnership with the NIH and being in partnership with, say, an industry. The goals of the NIH and those of clinical investigators are much the same: to improve health while trying to produce new knowledge. The investigator chooses the research project, and once the NIH approves it, the investigator receives funds. Neither partner, in most instances, expects that the research will lead to something that makes money.

When a clinical investigator collaborates with scientists in an industry, on the other hand, the people from the industry, not the investigator, usually choose the goal of the research. The goal may be a product, process, service, or something else, but whatever the goal, it will almost always be something that will eventually turn a profit. This does not make collaborations between industry and clinical departments impossibly awkward. On the contrary, such collaborations almost always benefit both partners. The industry usually has money to underwrite equipment and supplies and may also have an array of experts—chemists, physicists, model makers, mathematicians, and the like—who can help. In return, the clinical investigator can offer medical, as well as scientific, expertise. And if the project involves a new drug or some sort of medical device, the clinician can smooth the way for clinical trials.

The important point is that members of clinical departments, accustomed to having their research underwritten by NIH funds, will have to make adjustments if they turn to industry for support. But then, members of clinical departments these days are having to make adjustments of all sorts.

## Money, Departments, and Hospitals

Money, as much as anything else, determines the nature of the partnership between a clinical department and its hospital. These partnerships, under the best of circumstances, are love-hate relationships, as is usually true when two agencies with different goals must depend on each other for survival. Hospital administrators are driven crazy by members of clinical departments who fail to keep discharge summaries up to date, a mortal sin in the eyes of hospital accreditors. At the same time, members of clinical departments often accuse hospitals of short-changing them when, for instance, the hospital pays members of departments to read electrocardiograms, supervise clinical laboratories, or interpret pulmonary function tests.

Back in the 1960s, when I became responsible for the training program in cardiology at P and S, I found that the Presbyterian Hospital had several years earlier agreed to pay the salary of one of the four cardiology fellows, a sum of around $10,000. This was a godsend for the training program, because in those days, an extra salary was hard to come by. But in return for the salary, the four fellows were expected to read all the EKGs taken in the hospital. By the time I arrived, the number of EKGs had grown to 40,000 per year, a total that vastly exceeded the number needed for training. Whose fault was this unfortunate situation? No one's, really. The agreement between Cardiology and the hospital was struck at a time when Cardiology badly needed another fellow and the hospital badly needed people to read EKGs.

Then, at Stony Brook, we argued for months—ultimately years—over the amount that should be paid a hematologist from our department to supervise the hematology laboratory in the hospital. We went through a similar ordeal when we tried to agree on stipends for our pulmonary specialists, who supervised and interpreted pulmonary function tests. Disputes like these become especially awkward if the medical school runs the hospital, because faculty members may find themselves negotiating with other faculty members over payments.

Earning money is a good, not an evil, thing. Earned money is power, and in many schools this money is underwriting salaries, research, and dozens of other worthwhile things. But money becomes evil when the lure of high salaries makes people neglect teaching and research, the things universities are all about. This evil will plague chairs in the future, just as it has plagued them in the past. And there is no way, at the moment, to predict whether HMOs or other managed care systems will ameliorate the evil or make it worse.

## 15
## Departmental Quality and Departmental Reviews

When things are going well, when members of a department are contributing new knowledge to the literature and medical students are elbowing each other for spots in the training program, the quality of a department is evident. In this happy circumstance, a chair need only remember that maintaining quality is a never-ending process, a process that requires attention day after day. But when productivity falls or morale plummets, a review of some sort may be useful or necessary. There are many types of reviews to choose from. In this section, we shall look at four of them.

## Reviews

### Planning Sessions

The simplest, least-threatening type of review is a planning session in which the chair meets with the division chiefs (if the department has chiefs) or with senior department members (if it doesn't). The purpose of the meeting is to talk over how the department is going, to discuss sources of trouble, and to hammer out ways to get rid of them. Later, when the remedies have been polished and framed as projects, the chair presents the projects to the department for discussion.

In many departments, planning sessions are held at least once a year when things are going well. The sessions provide a first-class way to keep a department focused on quality and to head off trouble before it starts.

### Retreats

Retreats can be used in the same way as planning sessions, but retreats usually involve the entire department, not just the chair and senior people. And, like planning sessions, retreats are often held when things are going smoothly, when a department is prospering.

If a retreat is held when things are going badly, the chair will be in for a hard time. Young department members, especially the immature bad apples, will seize on the retreat as an opportunity to unload their complaints and indignation. Bennet and Figuli could, in fact, have been thinking about a chair at a retreat when they said the task of a chair "is not unlike the job of herding a bunch of frogs . . . a bastion of rampant individualism" (1993, xvi).

One tactic that may save a retreat from becoming a hand-wringing orgy is to start each part of the program with a summary of the things already accomplished, to stress the department's strengths in that area, rather than its weaknesses. The summary may help those who then offer comments to keep their remarks in perspective.

If, at the end of a retreat, a chair has a list of suggested remedies for present troubles and a list of new projects the department might undertake, the retreat can be counted a success.

## Divisional Reviews

Planning sessions and retreats can go a long way toward boosting morale and keeping the quality of a department high. Yet, a time will come when some sort of trouble will necessitate a more structured review. If the trouble is localized, restricted to a single division, for instance, the chair can carry out a divisional review without calling for outside help. This type of review entails first telling the division chief about the plan and then having a private information-gathering talk with each member of the division, spreading the talks over days or weeks. As the interviews go along, the cause of the trouble in the division usually becomes apparent. And after all of the members of the division have been interviewed, the chair meets with the chief and tells the chief—in general, anonymous terms—what the members have said. The chair then helps the chief find ways to eliminate the trouble.

The handful of divisional reviews I held or witnessed seemed to make things better, to lift the spirits of the people involved. Improvement occurred so consistently that I wondered whether it might be an example of the Hawthorne effect. Behavioral scientists use this term to describe the way people, asked to be the subjects of a project, may change before the project starts (Levine and Cohen 1974). Something about the protocol to be followed, or the location of the project, or the special attention paid the people who are to take part in the project, may be the explanation of these curious results.

An example comes from the work of Rashkis and Smarr (1957) who set out to test the effect of combinations of drugs in a group of patients with catatonic schizophrenia. The investigators transferred forty-eight patients from hospital wards to a research unit with special nurses, then made baseline measurements on the patients over a period of weeks. And during this period, before any of the drugs to be tested had been started, thirty-nine of the forty-eight patients improved. Moving the patients to the new unit and giving them special attention were thought to account for the improvement.

The Hawthorne effect got its name, incidentally, from a study carried out in the early part of this century at the Hawthorne plant of the Western Electric Company in Chicago. Things were going badly in the plant, and the management wanted to find out whether a change in working conditions would raise morale and productivity. Consultants were hired, and during an initial period, when the consultants were doing nothing but observing the workers, productivity increased. The consultants concluded that the rise in productivity came from the attention the workers received.

Whether or not the Hawthorne effect plays a role, divisional reviews are a useful intermediate step between informal reviews—like project-setting sessions and retreats—and formal, full-scale departmental reviews.

### Departmental Reviews

Periodic departmental reviews are mandated in some schools, and in these places, groups of outside experts visit departments according to a schedule set up in advance. The state of a department has nothing to do with the date the review gets going. The review takes place as scheduled, whether the department is doing well or floundering.

Nonmandated departmental reviews are different. They are one-shot affairs, arranged by the dean, when a department gets in trouble. I've never been sure these reviews accomplish much. Or, at least,

I've never been sure that they justify the time and energy they consume or the anxieties and animosities they generate. Members of an outside review committee may turn up new information, but will the information add much to what the dean already knows? Often, it seems to me, the chief function of the visitors is to give the dean ammunition—and to later shoulder part of the blame—when the dean fires the chair, something the dean had planned to do all along. *Because a full-scale, nonmandated review, carried out when a department is in trouble, is a review of the competence of the chair.*

In addition to borrowing the practice of reviews and audits from the world of business, hospitals and other health care agencies have, in recent years, borrowed something else: an assortment of management techniques meant to ensure the quality of medical care. Outcome reviews, for instance, have been used to evaluate the quality of surgical procedures, while process reviews have been used to determine whether the number of Caesarean sections performed is excessive.

Health care organizations have, in some instances, used a more comprehensive management system known as total quality control (TQC) to improve the efficiency of their operations. TQC was the invention of W. Edwards Deming (1982), a noted statistician and management consultant, who based his approach on the premise that building quality into every step of, say, a manufacturing process, will lead to lower costs, larger profits, and greater customer satisfaction. Deming stressed the importance of teamwork and communication, rather than competition and personal ambition. The Japanese seized on TQC and showed the premise to be sound. In fact, many people in that country credit TQC for the industrial success Japan has enjoyed the past few decades.

Recently, a group of cardiac surgeons, in a pioneering effort, launched a project to see whether TQC could be used to reduce mortality in open heart surgery (O'Connor et al. 1996). All twenty-three cardiac surgeons in Maine, New Hampshire, and Vermont, along with cardiologists, anesthesiologists, nurses, aides, and epidemiologists at the five medical centers where bypass surgery was being performed, took part in the project. Over a period of nine months, teams from each of the centers visited the other centers, watched pre-op and post-op procedures, as well as the operations, then compared what they saw with the way they did things at home. "There are hundreds of processes in cardiac surgery," O'Connor said. "There are dozens or hundreds of things people looked at or changed." And during the nine months the project was in progress, there were seventy-four fewer deaths than would have been expected. "This twenty-four percent reduction in the hospital mortality rate," the authors wrote, "was statistically significant (p .001) . . . and was temporally associated with the interventions" (841).

In connection with TQC, the Joint Commission on Accreditation of Healthcare Organizations had, until 1991, encouraged hospitals to use a management technique that resembled TQC, a technique called quality assurance (QA). Then the commission replaced QA with a new process called continuous quality improvement (CQI). CQI is, the commission said, a concept that "incorporates the strengths of QA, while broadening its scope, refining its approach to assessing and improving care, and dispensing with the negative connotations sometimes associated with QA." With this system, "care will be improved not by focusing primarily on outliers or bad apples but by looking at the complex series of activities that compose any key function in the hospital" (Joint Commission 1991, 7).

Now for a final point. In the 1960s and 1970s, medical schools, after slumbering for years, took renewed interest in the quality of their programs and installed reviews and evaluations in all sorts of areas. Stony Brook, then a new school, hired a director of medical education, whose sole duty was to review and evaluate teaching. The director would attend or tape a lecture, then later, in a private session, point out to the hapless lecturer the things he or she had done wrong. And students were enjoined to submit unsigned appraisals of all lectures and lecturers.

I managed to avoid the sessions with the director, but I could not avoid being handed the students' evaluations. One evaluation—two lines scrawled across a sheet of wrinkled paper—gave me the thought

I should like for my epitaph: "It takes genius to speak that slowly and still be confusing."

# 16
# The Effect of Distance on Unity

Chairs who try to instill a spirit of unity in their departments, especially departments with far-flung affiliates, will stub their toes on an immutable law: the greater the distance between people, the smaller the chance the people will meet and talk. The meaning of the law is obvious, but the pervasive nature of the law is not so obvious. It applies to people working only a few yards from each other just as it does to people working at places that are miles apart.

The effect of the law at short distances came to light when T. J. Allen (1970) studied the relation between communication and distance in a building filled with men and women working on a research project. He recorded the frequency with which the researchers consulted each other, then plotted the frequency as a function of the distance between their desks. As the distance widened, the frequency plummeted.

"The proportion of people with whom an individual communicates," Allen wrote, "decays with the square of the distance outward from the focal person." This fact, he said, was not too surprising. But it was surprising, he added, that the probability of communication reached a low, fixed level at about twenty-five yards. This suggests that a person may not talk any more frequently to a colleague who is twenty-five yards away than to a colleague who is miles away. After Allen got similar results in two other studies, he concluded, "the effect appears to be general and independent of the technical work being performed" (18).

As might be expected, the frequency of communication is also diminished if people have desks on different floors. With another researcher, Alan R. Fustfeld, Allen showed that vertical separation jeopardizes communication at least as much as horizontal separation, and that elevators do not seem to change the situation in the case of one or two floors (1975, 156).

Communication becomes even more difficult when people are located in different buildings. At a VA hospital where I worked, the director's office was in an administration building that sat two hundred yards away from the hospital. As a consequence, we seldom saw the director, except at infrequent, formal meetings. Hence, there was little opportunity to get to know the person. Most of the time, the directors let us know their wishes by sending us memorandums. These documents—cold, formal, and laced with government prose—gave the impression of commands from on high and imposed a terrible strain on collegiality. I served under four different directors, and the effect of the memos was the same with each one. The root trouble was the distance that made the directives necessary, not the personalities of those holding the office.

In addition to distance, certain features of a building may impede communication. Allen termed them "nuisance factors" and cited corners and stairways as examples. When structures like these make the path from one desk to another 25 to 50 percent longer than the straight line between two points, the probability of communication, Allen found, again falls to a low, fixed level. A friend once told me that he seldom had a chance to talk to the chair of his department, though I learned when I visited my friend that his office was just down the hall from the chair's. The trouble, I've always suspected, was that the chair's door opened onto the hall, while my friend's door was around a corner, on a short, dead-end stem that branched off of the hall. Corners can, as mentioned, block easy talk.

The location of a person's desk is important also, and this is especially true in the case of the boss. In a law firm, for instance, when a partner becomes head, it is customary for the partner to move to the corner office, the one with the best view. Allen and Fustfeld question the wisdom of the move and have this to say: "One thing is certain: the head of an organization who wants to keep in close touch with what is going on must resist the temptation to locate in the corner with the best view. The center of the building is the best place. This will minimize average separation from his office and the location of groups reporting to him. Otherwise, he is going to be farther from some groups than from others, with a corresponding degradation in communication" (156).

Are there structures that encourage communication, rather than impede it? Yes. The photocopier, in our department, brought people together to talk and gossip, as the town pump did in frontier days. The coffee maker played a similar role.

And are there events that promote exchanges between department members? The answer again is yes. Getting everyone in the department together for wine and cheese on Friday afternoons worked well for us. And exercises like grand rounds, held in an auditorium or amphitheater, promote communication between faculty members, in addition to keeping them up to date.

The most damaging effect of distance for a clinical department lies in the relation of the affiliates to the home base. Here, the frequency of communication often depends more on travel time than on distance. And as travel time increases, the chance that people from different places will meet and talk becomes vanishingly small.

Annual meetings, rotated between the home department and the affiliates, can help. So can monthly meetings of an executive committee, rotated in the same way. Inviting people from affiliates to teach at the school has an especially good effect. And, if at all practical, an exchange of physicians for teaching rounds is a marvelous way to make faculty members from affiliates feel they belong.

In view of the foregoing points, it is, I think, fair to say that chairs who try to bring unity to their departments, who try to bind together the home base and the affiliates, have the odds stacked against them. Distance can be a malignant, intractable foe.

# 17
# Legal Issues

My introduction to legal issues in medical schools came shortly after I was appointed chair. I had gone to a meeting in Washington, D.C., and had run into a friend who headed a clinical department in a southern university. When I asked how things were going, he grimaced and said, "It's hard to tell." Then he told this story.

He had noticed that a chief and members of the chief's division were spending large amounts of unauthorized time in the clinical practice area. So my friend walked into the chief's office one afternoon and asked the chief what he was doing with the money he and his colleagues were collecting from the extra clinical practice. The chief waffled, then promised to deliver a full account of the income. My friend left the chief and walked back to his own office. He had just arrived when the telephone rang. It was the chief's secretary, who said, "My boss has had second thoughts about sending you an account of the money. He suggests you speak to his attorney."

I was shaken. I had never heard of faculty members speaking to each other through attorneys, nor could I imagine a chief sending such a message to a chair.

A short time later, I had another lesson in the legal aspects of medicine. A neurosurgeon on our staff, a man known for his conservative, careful work, had been asked to consult on one of our patients. An hour after the neurosurgeon left, I dropped by to see the patient, a soft-spoken, elderly man who single-handedly took care of an ailing wife. The man, sitting in bed behind drawn curtains, was in tears. "The neurosurgeon told me," he said, "that unless I have an operation on my head, I will die. If I do have the operation, there's only a 50 percent chance that I will live through it. And if I come out alive, there's a good chance I'll be partly paralyzed."

I went to see the neurosurgeon, to ask why he had spoken to the patient in such brutal terms. "My malpractice premium just went up to $80,000," he said. "If I give a patient hope and something bad happens, the patient will sue and my premium will go higher." I was shaken a second time, for I had not yet learned, back in the early 1970s, that fear of a lawsuit could affect the way a physician talks to patients.

A new chair these days will smile at my naïveté. He or she will most likely have heard of a lawsuit between faculty members and will certainly know about malpractice suits. A new chair may also have heard about a half-dozen other legal issues that sometimes surface in academic deprtments (see Figuli 1993).

I'm going to talk about malpractice and then about two issues that every chair must know how to handle. One is discrimination in hiring and firing, and the other is harassment. Then I shall talk about noninclusive language, a topic that, while not a legal issue, is so closely related to sexual discrimination that it is, I believe, worth mentioning.

## Malpractice

Nowadays, we hear more about malpractice than about other legal issues in medical schools. Yet clinical chairs are, in my experience, seldom involved in these suits in any direct way. A chair may offer support and sympathy if a clinician in the department is sued, but the principals in the suit will, in all likelihood, be the clinician and the clinician's attorney, the patient and the patient's attorney, the attorney for the hospital, and, in some instances, the attorney for the medical school or practice plan. The chair may, of ocurse, be involved if he or she had a hand in the care of the patient in question, or if, as happened in my department, the plaintiff happens to be a member of the family of someone in the department. In the latter instance, the role of the chair will be to try to repair the damage that such incidents inflict on a departmental faculty.

Chairs are also seldom involved in malpractice suits against interns or residents. A chair is responsible for selecting these young men and women, for training them to practice good medicine, and for providing support if they get into trouble, but the salaries of interns and residents and the premiums for their malpractice insurace are usually paid by hospitals. Hence, an intern or resident accused of malpractice is more apt to be defended by a hospital attorney than by an attorney from a department or school.

## Discrimination in Hiring and Firing

In contrast to their relative immunity in matters connected with malpractice, chairs are directly responsible for observing the laws and regulations that govern the hiring and firing of staff members. Title VII of the Civil Rights Act of 1964 makes it unlawful for a chair, or other employer, to base a decision to hire or fire on a person's race, color, religion, creed, sex, or nationality. In the years that have gone by since Title VII was enacted, other laws, especially the Civil Rights Act of 1991, have further spelled out the steps an employer must take to guard against discriminating.

Fortunately, medical schools and universities now have experts a chair can turn to for help. At Stony Brook, for instance, we have an office for human resources in the medical school, a second office in the hospital, and a third office in the nonmedical part of the university. These offices, with their resident experts, are backed up by full-time attorneys. The university also gives each chair a thick notebook entitled *Search and Selection Guidelines*, which, in addition to detailing the rules that govern hiring and firing, contains practical tools, like model letters for offering a job to a candidate and for notifying those candidates who were not selected, and lists of permissible and impermissible questions to guide chairs when interviewing candidates. So, modern-day chairs have a variety of resources to help them avoid discriminating.

## Harassment

Harassment, like discrimination in hiring and firing, is the direct concern of every chair. This is especially true of sexual harassment, a problem that has in recent years received nationwide attention. According to Elizabeth Fox-Genovese, author of *Feminism Is Not the Story of My Life* (1996), "sexual harassment suits have multiplied during the past five years, especially in the colleges and universities that have so prided themselves on the diversity of their work force and their openness to women" (A40–A41).

Justice Ruth Bader Ginsburg offered a definition of sexual harassment in her first appearance as a justice of the Supreme Court. The case being heard that morning was about sexual harassment, and the opposing attorneys were arguing over the definition of such terms as *reasonable woman* and *reasonable act.* Justice Ginsburg broke in and "asked why sexual harassment should not be defined simply as conduct that on the basis of an employee's sex makes it more difficult for one person than another to perform the job. 'How about just saying that?' " she proposed (Greenhouse 1993). This definition, it seems to me, is an impressively clear and useful guide.

Examples of the types of conduct that experts warn against are verbal abuse, unnecessary touching, demands for sexual favors either by implication or through threats, and making such favors a condition for employment, advancement, or admission to an academic program. The ramifications of these types of behavior have become so important that our university, like most others, I suspect, has a special office, staffed by experts, to help chairs and other faculty members deal with them.

Noninclusive language is connected to sexual discrimination in a subtle but definite way. The use of such language in scholarly works by men, for instance, is often viewed as an attempt to discriminate against women. A number of books have been written on how to avoid sexist writing, but the best source of instruction, in my view, is the fourth edition of William Zinsser's small, indispensable book *On Writing Well: An Informal Guide to Writing Nonfiction* (1990). In the introduction to this fourth edition, Zinsser mentions his realization that he needed to remove the sexist language he had used in the first three editions; and then, on pages 117–20, he tells the reader how he went about doing this. Studying what he says will help any writer, but still more helpful is a side-by-side comparison with the third edition of the book, if you can lay hands on one. This exercise will convince anyone that a book can be made to read as smoothly with inclusive nouns and pronouns as with their sexist counterparts.

When a chair has to handle matters relating to malpractice, hiring, firing, or harassment, he or she will often have to turn to experts for help. But even with an expert next door, the best defense against wrongs is, as everyone knows, to keep them from happening. Since this will not always be possible, a chair should keep detailed written records of all performance evaluations and untoward incidents. At the same time, chairs should remember that common sense, good faith, and collegiality are still the best tools for handling incidents that might give rise to legal challenges, just as these tools have always been.

# 18
# A Conviction, an Attitude, and a Blessing

A chair—or any other medical or nonmedical leader—will have the best chance for happiness if he or she has a conviction, an attitude, and a blessing. The conviction is the knowledge that, despite enjoying the job, he or she could be just as happy doing something else. The something else may be research or medical practice or something never tried before. Either way, nothing so prepares a chair to make hard decisions as knowing that another job would bring as much pleasure and satisfaction as leading a department. The importance of this point was brought home to me by S. Marsh Tenney, the friend already mentioned: "Chairs and deans must be prepared to take positions that may cost them their jobs."

The attitude a chair should try to cultivate may charitably be called self-delusion or, uncharitably, arrogance. When a chair sits home and reflects on the way his or her job is going, the chair should be able to say he or she is doing the job about as well as most people could. Here, chairs must use common sense and compare themselves to contemporaries in similar jobs. Measuring themselves against an Osler, Halstead, or Christian is self-defeating. They were great, without question, but great in different jobs, in different times. Reassuring themselves will be difficult for chairs, just as it's difficult for everyone. "Deep down in his heart," Mark Twain said, "no man much respects himself."

The third need of a chair—the blessing—is a colleague the chair can talk to, confide in, and bounce ideas against. Ideally, the colleague should be smarter than the chair, a person with a fine and complex mind, who has a feel for people, understands human behavior, and, above all else, holds sacred anything said in confidence.

But even when chairs have the conviction, the attitude, and the blessing, their grip on happiness will be tenuous, the tie to their job a slender thread. The black dog of self-doubt will trot along behind them, just as it trots behind leaders everywhere. George Long knew these things a century ago when he wrote about the great emperor Antoninus: "The best and the bravest have moments of doubt and weakness, but if they are the best and the bravest, they rise again from their depression by recurring to first principles" (1909, 330–31).

# III

# Solving Problems

## 19
## Karl Popper: Solving Problems with the Conscious Mind

Whether serving as academic leader or department manager, a chair spends more time grappling with problems than doing anything else. Some of the problems are unique to the chair's specialty, but most are the type that every chair, at one time or another, will have to handle. Although dozens of books and articles have been written about problems, none that I have read compares with the pioneering works of Karl Popper, Henri Poincaré, and René Descartes. Popper told us how the conscious mind deals with problems, Poincaré showed us how the subconscious helps, and Descartes gave us four rules for bringing a problem under attack. So, in the next three sections, I shall briefly review what Popper, Poincaré, and Descartes said. And since the ideas of each man grew out of his work, his education, or his personal experience, I shall include, for each of the three, a short biographical sketch.

Popper was born in Vienna in 1902. He studied mathematics, science, philosophy, and physics in secondary school, then, after graduating, taught for several years. In 1936, sensing that Hitler planned to seize Austria, Popper left his homeland and went to New Zealand. He taught philosophy at the University of New Zealand, then, when the war ended, left New Zealand for England and joined the staff of the London School of Economics. Throughout the time from 1936 until his death a few years ago, Popper published extraordinary insights on a variety of topics, including science, historicism, and Marxism.

Popper's work, said Bryan Magee, "unlike that of so many contemporary philosophers, has a notably *practical* effect on people who are influenced by it: it changes the way they do their own work, and in this and other respects, changes their lives" (1973, 2). Certainly, this was true for me after my long-time friend and mentor S. Marsh Tenney introduced me to Popper twenty years ago. And a comment Marsh made about his own experience of Popper's work was true for me also: "It must be admitted that Popper's message contained in *Objective Knowledge* and in *The Logic of Scientific Discovery* requires intense concentration and perseverance, but of inestimable help is Bryan Magee's *Karl Popper*, a book that analyzes succinctly the essence of Popper's philosophy" (1993, 51). Magee's book, in my opinion, should be near the top of the reading list of every chair.

Though Popper wrote on diverse topics, a theme that pervades many of his books and papers is the importance of problem solving. "All organisms," he wrote, "are constantly, day and night, engaged in problem-solving; and so are all those evolutionary sequences of organisms—the phyla which begin with the most primitive forms and of which the now living organisms are the latest members" (Magee, 51).

Popper took as a first principle the belief that we seldom solve a problem in any complete or permanent way. Instead, our solution simply converts the problem to a new and different form. The new form will suffice for the moment, but it, too, may have to be changed at some time in the future. Hence, a typical problem has a past history, a train of events that led to the problem's present state, and will have a future, as solutions are put in place, then modified.

We convert a problem to a new form, Popper said, through a sequence resembling that shown below:

$$P1 \rightarrow TS \rightarrow EE \rightarrow P2,$$

where P1 is the initial problem, TS is a trial solution, EE is an error-eliminating step taken to test the merit of the trial solution, refine the trial solution, or compare the worth of one trial solution to that of another, and P2 is the problem converted to its new form. (Magee, 60)

To illustrate this process, let us suppose a dean decides the hospital census is too low and tells the chair of obstetrics and gynecology to increase the number of patients on the OB-GYN service. The chair's problem (P1) is a department with too few patients. The chair's task is to find a way to increase the number.

One obvious way (TS) would be to require all members of the department to enlarge their practices and admit more patients. To test (EE) the merit of this solution, the chair makes an estimate of the number of hours that would be required to add new patients to a practice, to admit some of the patients, and to then take care of them. If the number of hours is large, the chair realizes that these hours could come only from those being used for research. So, if the chair chooses this solution, the problem will change from a department with too few patients (P1) to a department with enough patients but a diminished capability for research (P2). The trial solution has modified the problem, not abolished it. And the chair has been reminded of a lesson taught by Machiavelli: "one inconvenience cannot be avoided except at the risk of being exposed to another" (101–2).

If P2 is unacceptable, the chair searches for a new trial solution, then tests that one to see what new form of the problem it will produce. The process continues until the chair finds the solution that will increase the census and have the least-damaging side effects.

The problem of too few patients is typical of the problems all chairs carry around in their heads. For some of the problems, they are seeking trial solutions, for others, error-eliminating steps to test the trial solutions they have come up with. And for still others, they are pondering ways to implement the solutions they have decided to put in place. Chairs work unceasingly on problems. Yet, many of the problems they tackle will persist, no matter what they do.

# 20
# Henri Poincaré:
# Solving Problems with
# the Subconscious Mind

Whereas Popper wrote mostly about the conscious mind, Henri Poincaré wrote about the role the subconscious plays in problem solving and creativity. Poincaré was eminently qualified to do this, because his own creative output was formidable. In thirty-four years Poincaré published more than thirty books on mathematical physics and celestial mechanics and nearly five hundred memoirs on mathematics (Newman 1956, 2:1375).

Poincaré was born in Nancy, France, in 1854. He attended the Nancy Polytechnic School and the Nancy School of Mines, then earned a doctorate in mathematical sciences at the University of Paris. With doctorate in hand, Poincaré joined the faculty of the University of Caen and during the next few years carried out research of such high quality that he was elected to the Academy of Sciences at the age of thirty-two. The academician who nominated him declared that Poincaré had settled questions that in the past were unimagined.

Early on, Poincaré developed an interest in creativity, and he apparently maintained the interest for the rest of his life. He wrote a long essay on creativity, and though he focused on creative thought in mathematics, his insights apply to creative thought in any field (Poincaré 1952, 46). "It is time to penetrate further," Poincaré began, "and to see what goes on in the very soul of the mathematician.

For this purpose I think I cannot do better than recount my personal recollections. Only I am going to confine myself to relating how I wrote my first treatise on Fuchsian functions" (52–53).

Then Poincaré told this story. For two weeks he had tried to prove that certain mathematical expressions, which he called Fuchsian functions, were unique. Each day he had sat at his desk, sometimes for several hours, testing one combination after another, but without success. Then one night, after drinking black coffee, he slept fitfully. "A host of ideas kept surging in my head; I could almost feel them jostling one another, until two of them coalesced, so to speak, to form a stable combination. When next morning came, I had established the existence of one class of Fuchsian functions, those that are derived from the hypergeometric series. I had only to verify the results" (52–53).

Shortly afterward, Poincaré left Caen to go on a field trip sponsored by the School of Mines. In one of the villages they visited, as he stepped up into the bus, he had an insight: the transformations he had used to define the Fuchsian functions were identical with those of non-Euclidean geometry. "I made no verification," he said, "and had no time to do so, since I took up the conversation again as soon as I sat down . . . , but I felt absolute certainty" (53).

"These sudden inspirations," Poincaré wrote, "are never produced . . . except after some days of voluntary efforts which appeared absolutely fruitless, in which one thought one had accomplished nothing." Then after the inspiration, Poincaré continues, there's need for a second period of conscious work, a period in which the person shapes the inspiration and examines its meaning (56).

But what happens during the period of subconscious thought? Poincaré offers the following analogy:

If I may be permitted a crude comparison, let us represent the future elements of our combinations as something resembling Epicurus's hooked atoms. When the mind is in complete repose these atoms are immovable; they are, so to speak, attached to the wall.

On the other hand, during a period of apparent repose . . . some of them are detached from the wall and set in motion. They plough through space in all directions, like a swarm of gnats. . . . Their mutual collisions may then produce new combinations.

The purpose of the preliminary conscious work, he said, is to shake the atoms and unhook them from the wall. "We think we have accomplished nothing, when we have stirred up the elements in a thousand different ways. . . . The liberated atoms will then experience collisions" until the right combination is found (60–62).

Rudolph Flesch collected comments from people who had learned to rely on the subconscious for help in solving problems. One was Louis Bromfield, who wrote,

One of the most helpful discoveries I made long ago in common with some other writers, is that there is a part of the mind, which the psychologists call the *subconscious*, that works while you are sleeping or even while you are relaxing or are engaged in some other task far removed from writing. I have found it possible to train this part of the mind to do a pretty organized job. Very often I have awakened in the morning to find a problem of technique, or plot, or character, which had long been troubling me, completely solved while I had been sleeping. (Flesch 1949, 56)

A second person whose comments Flesch noted was Bertrand Russell, who said, "I have found that if I have to write upon some very difficult topic, the best plan is to think about it with very great intensity—the greatest intensity of which I am capable—for a few hours or days, and at the end of that time give orders, so to speak, that the work is to proceed underground. After some time I return consciously to the topic and find the work has been done" (56).

Some say that physical activity helps shake insights loose. Naguib Mahfouz, winner of the 1988 Nobel Prize in literature, rises early each morning and walks the streets of Cairo, writes Alan Cowell (1988), who interviewed him for the *New York Times*. The walk—which lasts about ninety minutes—takes Mahfouz from his suburban home to the Ali Baba coffee house in downtown Cairo, where he meets friends, talks, and reads the newspapers. "The walk is the important thing," the author told Cowell. "I can sleep on a problem without finding a solution. But when I'm walking, an idea will come to me."

There are two other points to be made about the subconscious. One is that it enables us to work on multiple problems at the same time. While one is applying conscious thought to one problem, the subconscious is processing others. The second point, in Flesch's words, is that "bright new ideas are always combinations of old ones." And more often than not, these combinations come from the subconscious mind.

Chairs are utterly dependent on the subconscious. Without the ability to work on multiple problems simultaneously, they would drown. And Poincaré was right, I suspect, when he said that the subconscious can, in a short time, make more different combinations than the conscious mind can make in a lifetime.

## 21
## René Descartes: Solving Problems by Using Four Rules

Unlike Popper and Poincaré, who were interested in problem solving generally, René Descartes focused on a single problem: how to distinguish truth from untruth. And as a step toward making the distinction, Descartes devised four rules which, he believed, would enable him to do this. The rules were tailored to meet Descartes's specific need, yet they were so general that they turned out to be useful for attacking problems of any sort.

Descartes was born in Touraine in 1596, when Europe was emerging from its medieval past and embracing a new age of reason and enlightenment. At the age of eight, Descartes entered La Fleche, a prestigious Jesuit school, where he was placed in a special group of students "not subject to the stricter discipline of the rest; for . . . Descartes was allowed by the rector, Father Charlet, to lie in bed in the morning—a habit which he maintained all his life, and which he regarded as above all conducive to intellectual profit and comfort" (Mahaffy 1969, 11–12).

Descartes studied the humanities for five and one half years, then science and mathematics for two and one half more; yet, when he had completed his studies, he was, he said, "not learned but ignorant."

The belief that he was ignorant led Descartes to think more and more about the way he had been educated. He began to have doubts about the scholastic philosophy his professors had taught him. He doubted, for instance, that relying on the authority of Aristotle was a good idea, and he agreed with Francis Bacon that scientists should make their own observations, rather than accept what Aristotle or anyone else had said. So Descartes "resolved no longer to seek any other science than the knowledge of myself, or of the great book of the world" (1910, 10). And thus began his search for truth.

Descartes wanted, above all, to keep the search simple, and he believed that the aforementioned four rules would "prove perfectly sufficient for me, provided I took the firm and unwavering resolution never in a single instance to fail in observing them."

> The *first* was never to accept anything for true which I did not clearly know to be such; that is to say, carefully to avoid precipitancy and prejudice, and to comprise nothing more in my judgment than what was presented to my mind so clearly and distinctly as to exclude all ground of doubt.
>
> The *second*, to divide each of the difficulties under examination into as many parts as possible, and as might be necessary for its adequate solution.
>
> The *third*, to conduct my thoughts in such order that, by commencing with objects the simplest and easiest to know, I might ascend by little and little, and, as it were, step by step, to the knowledge of the more complex; assigning in thought a certain order even to those ob-

jects which in their own nature do not stand in a relation of antecedence and sequence.

And the *fourth* is to make enumerations so complete, and reviews so general, that I might be assured that nothing was omitted. (17–18)

Mortimer Adler and Seymour Cain (1963) caught the essence of the rules in the following shortened versions:

1. Accept nothing as true unless it is presented to the mind so clearly and distinctly that it cannot be doubted.
2. Divide each problem into as many parts as possible, in order to reach the most adequate solution.
3. Proceed in gradual order from the simplest and most easily understood objects to knowledge of the most complex.
4. Make complete and comprehensive surveys and checks to ensure that nothing has been omitted. (160)

"Descartes was convinced," Adler and Cain said, "that with these few and simple rules he had arrived at a method for acquiring knowledge in all things which was comparable to that by which geometricians arrive at demonstrable and certain truths" (160).

Descartes applied his four rules to studies of—among other things—optics, the solar system, and mathematics, especially geometry. Then in 1637, at the age of forty-one, he wrote a long essay entitled *Discourse on the Method of Properly Guiding the Reason in the Research of Truth in the Sciences.* The work was a record, a personal journal, of how the four rules had helped him keep his thinking straight.

Descartes had no interest in arguing the merits of his method or imposing it on others. His design, he said, was "not to teach the method which everyone should follow in order to promote the good conduct of his reason, but only to show in what manner I have endeavoured to conduct my own." Despite Descartes's inclination to keep the method for himself, the *Discourse* had far-reaching consequences. This was true because Descartes had placed at the center of his system the question, "What is the origin of human knowledge?", a question that had plagued philosophers everywhere. Descartes had, in addition, shown that this question, like most others, cannot be answered satisfactorily without also asking, "How do I know?" Descartes's approach touched a second subject of broad importance: the belief that a person seeking truth had to start with doubt, not faith—a belief the all-powerful medieval Church fiercely opposed (Hart 1987, 334–35).

Descartes worked in Holland for twenty years, then moved to Stockholm when Christina, queen of Sweden, invited him to be her tutor. But once there, Descartes found the Stockholm winter unbearably harsh. Also, James R. Newman tells us, "the Queen shattered the unhappy man's lifelong routine by requiring him to instruct her daily at 5 in the morning" (1956, 1:236). Descartes withstood the rigors of the weather and the schedule for four months, then he contracted pneumonia and died.

Dozens of books have been published on problems and how to solve them. The authors have all, in one way or another, repeated what Descartes said. They have had to repeat him, because the four rules Descartes devised more than three centuries ago have turned out to be bedrock principles for solving problems in any age.

# 22

# The Connection between Problem Solving, Writing, and Thinking

According to William Zinsser, a person sitting down to write is a person sitting down to solve a problem. "It may be a problem of where to obtain the facts or how to organize the material. It may be a problem of approach or attitude, tone or style. Whatever it is, it has to be confronted and solved" (1990, 59).

Conversely, a person having trouble with a problem should sit down and write about it. When the person pours out thoughts onto paper, possible solutions invariably come to mind. The solutions may be impractical; they may not include the one eventually chosen. But possible solutions beget possible solutions, and these, in turn, lead to a solution that will work.

In short, we solve problems when we're writing, and we use writing to solve problems. Writing and problem solving are inextricably linked.

A friend of mine made the following entry in his journal a few weeks after becoming head of a large clinical department in a northeastern school:

> The job is awesome, but I'm lucky in that I have a powerful tool for solving problems. It entails: sitting down and framing a precise statement of what I think the problem is; writing out my thoughts about the problem, letting the words tumble onto the pages in majestic disarray; revising my statement of the problem if the writing has changed my understanding of it; dividing the problem into parts, if this is advantageous; listing solutions that come to mind; writing a short discussion of each solution, including—when indicated—a table of advantages and disadvantages; letting the solutions incubate a day or two; getting the opinions of others about the different possibilities; and eventually choosing the solution which appears to have the most beneficial features and the fewest drawbacks.
>
> Once I've made the choice, I get a notebook and list the steps I'll have to take to implement the solution, keeping in mind that many small steps are better than a few big ones. I then start taking the steps—chipping off small hunks—whenever I have spare minutes. I return to my notebook every weekend, to record my progress, to add information I've picked up, and to decide about the next steps to take. It's a great system. It has solved such problems as how to govern the department, how to handle appointments and promotions, and how to teach clinical clerks.

Writing about a problem has much to recommend it. For instance, there is a limit to how many solutions one can hold in one's head. Elstein, Shulman, and Sprafka wrote that in making diagnoses, a special form of problem solving, "the size of the set of hypotheses being explored . . . is usually around four or five and appears to have an upper bound of about six or seven. These estimates are entirely consistent with other estimates of memory capacity for complex material" (279). Hence, when we think about solutions without writing them down, we're limited to about half a dozen possibilities.

A second advantage has to do with the precision the mind displays when we write about a problem we're trying to solve. Zinsser reports that he was "struck by one of the miracles of the cognitive process— that the act of writing will summon from the buried past exactly what we need exactly when we need it" (1988, 55).

Writing things down is also an effective way to set goals. This would be expected, since setting a goal is the same as creating a problem: the goal-setter must find a way to overcome the obstacles that stand between him and the goal. So the goal-setter starts by writing down the goal, just as the problem-solver starts by writing down the problem.

In addition to using writing to solve problems and set goals, chairs can use writing to find out what they think. Because it is only when we get our thoughts laid out on paper that we can know our true opinions and our reasons for holding them. "Very often," said Joseph Epstein, editor of *The American Scholar*, "the familiar essayist—or at least this one—does not know what he thinks until he has finished writing about it" (1979, viii).

Zinsser called this kind of writing *exploratory*, "writing that enables us to discover what we want to say" (1988, 56). Writing of any kind, Zinsser said, "compels us by the repeated effort of language to go after . . . thoughts and to organize them and present them clearly. It forces us to keep asking, 'Am I saying what I want to say?' Very often the answer is 'No' " (45).

The process works like a zero-error feedback loop, a loop that feeds the image of the written words back to the brain, where the words are compared to the thought that gave rise to them. If the words and thought differ, the writer tries to bring the difference to zero by changing the words. But this process—in a crisp and awe-some way—often reveals flaws in the thought itself. So the writer sharpens the thought, and then, in iterative fashion, repeats the process until the thought is straight and the written words reflect it. With complex issues, it may take repeated attempts, over days, weeks, or months, to bring the difference to zero.

These error-correcting steps resemble those a medical student takes when she listens to a heart, then tries to sketch the sounds on paper. She listens, removes her stethoscope, draws what she hears, and then, just to be sure she's got it right, listens again. This time, she hears something slightly different, so she corrects her sketch. And on and on until she believes she's heard the sounds right, and her sketch accurately depicts them. She has, so far as she can tell, brought the difference between sounds and sketch to zero.

"All erroneous ideas," wrote Luc de Clapiers, Marquis de Vauve-nargues, two centuries ago, "would perish of their own accord if expressed clearly" (Seldes 1985, 430). Writing is the only way to obtain such clarity. And the clarity comes through the zero-error principle.

Writing not only straightens our thoughts but also helps us understand. Zinsser mentions this when reminiscing about what writing can do: "I thought of how often as a writer I had made clear some subject I had previously known nothing about by just putting one sentence after another—by reasoning my way in sequential steps to its meaning. I thought of how often the act of writing even the simplest document—a letter, for instance—had clarified my half-formed ideas. Writing and thinking and learning were the same process" (1988, viii–ix).

Writing to understand can help leaders in another way. If they write regularly about their jobs, they will come to see them in a new light and slowly but steadily change the way they do their work.

Finally, writing to understand can be used to help break the grip of a depression, for writing about one's worries helps bring them into the open, just as they are brought into the open by talking them over with an old and trusted friend. "It is a great human truth," wrote Rabbi Joshua Roth Liebman, "that when we unlock our hearts to any sympathetic listener, our burdens often take wings" (1946, 37).

The effect of bringing things into the open may help explain the results obtained by Dr. Paulette Selmi and her colleagues, who studied the response of depressed patients to three types of therapy. Twelve patients were treated by a therapist; twelve had regular sessions with an "interactive" psychotherapeutic computer program; and twelve had no treatment at all. After six weeks, the untreated patients were unchanged. Those who saw a therapist "showed significant improvement." And those who used the computer program showed as much improvement as those treated by a therapist. The computer program, if nothing else, brought troubles into the open, just as writing and talking do.

Chairs, then, can use exploratory writing to find out what they think, to examine their opinions, and to help them understand their jobs. And they can, if they need and wish, use writing to ease the pain of depression and despair.

## 23
# Using Writing to Look Inside a Person's Head

Just as writing can reveal one's own thoughts and opinions, so can the writing of others provide a look inside their heads. I had suspected this before I became a chair, and had, from time to time, tried to correlate the writing of people I knew with their traits, habits, and patterns of thought. I'd come to believe that muddled sentences reflected careless thinking; that using the passive voice, except in scientific journals, might be an attempt to dodge responsibility; that the frequent use of compound sentences signaled an inability to separate the important from the trivial; and that writing peppered with exclamations suggested naïveté.

So I was cheered when I picked up the *New York Times* one morning during the 1988 presidential campaign and found an op-ed piece by a man who used people's writing to help him judge them. The man was Ladd Hamilton, former editor of the *Lewiston Morning Tribune*, in Lewiston, Idaho, who complained of not seeing examples of the candidates' writing "untouched by editors or image makers." Hamilton observed that it made a difference whether a candidate wrote in the active or passive voice or was "willing to split an infinitive." It was "the difference between knowing and not knowing how a candidate thinks."

Off hand, it would seem simpler to judge people by what they say, since people talk more than they write. Reasoned talk is, of course, a useful index. But casual talk gives few clues to serious thinking, because such talk is usually first-draft stuff. We speak before we've revised and sharpened. Points made in casual conversation may or may not reflect how we really feel.

Now, to end this brief section with a story about two men, two words, and two notes. André Cournand, although born and educated in France, used the English language beautifully. Yet, a few English words gave him trouble, and two of those words were *deceive* and *disappoint.*

This became important when Richard Bing came to New York to give a Harvey Lecture. On the afternoon before the lecture, Dr. Bing visited his old friend Cournand and explained that after his talk he would have to rush off to catch a plane and wouldn't have a chance to see him. He asked Cournand to write and tell him whether he thought the lecture went all right. Dr. Cournand said he would.

The next morning, Dr. Cournand penned this note to Dr. Bing: "Dear Richard, You deceived me. Yours, André." A few days later, this note came back: "Dear André, It is better to deceive a man than a woman. Yours, Richard."

# IV

## Teaching and Research

### 24
### Teaching at the Bedside

On a bright September morning many years ago, I went on rounds with an older friend, a physician admired for his skill as a bedside teacher. I wanted to watch him teach, to find out why students, interns, and residents often said he was the best teacher anywhere. My friend, a senior professor at the Boston University School of Medicine, would be making rounds on Evans 4, the teaching service of the Department of Medicine at the Massachusetts Memorial Hospitals. He would have with him two interns, two residents, and six clinical clerks. And when we had all assembled, my friend led us into the room of a patient, a middle-aged man who greeted us with a smile and a good-morning. At first glance, the man looked healthy. Then we saw that his skin was yellow.

My friend introduced himself, then introduced each of us. He told the patient that we were on teaching rounds and asked him if he minded if we discussed his illness. "No, I don't mind," the man said. "I might learn something. More important, you might find out why I'm sick."

My friend thanked him, then turned to one of the clerks and asked, "Can you, from what you see, tell us what problem we should tackle first?"

"The jaundice," the young man replied.

"And what, do you suppose, could be causing it?"

"Liver disease."

"What questions should we ask?"

"Do you drink?"

The man broke in, "Never. I don't like the stuff."

My friend then asked the clerk, "Does this alter your diagnosis?"

"In a sense it does. I'm still thinking about liver disease, but liver disease in a man who doesn't drink."

"What should we do next?"

"Ask about hepatitis."

How simple, I thought. My friend teaches by asking questions, just like the rest of us do. But after we had finished our visit with the jaundiced man and had seen other patients, it dawned on me that there was more to my friend's questions than was evident at first. Even though he phrased the questions in all sorts of ways, most of the questions asked, in effect, "What, in your opinion, . . . ?" Occasionally, he would ask for a fact, as in, "What's the normal range for serum sodium?" But when he asked for a fact, he'd turn from the clerk and ask all of us. This teacher asked mostly for opinions. His questions were an invitation to reason, not an inquisition.

In looking back I realize that my friend's approach to analyzing a patient's condition resembled the one Philip Tumulty later published in his book, *The Effective Clinician* (1973). Tumulty thought that the way to start thinking about a patient was to (1) pick an abnormality to puzzle over, preferably something from the history or physical examination, (2) pick something that looked as if it could be central to the illness, (3) be sure the something was real, and (4) avoid things that had a large number of causes (e.g., "tired feeling") and those that had so few causes they limited thought (e.g., an increased level of glutamine in the blood).

Once my friend had started a dialogue with a clerk or intern, he focused his attention—more often than not—on the best next step. Should we do this test or that? How would our thinking change if the test were positive? Negative?

I think my friend was using something like Popper's problem-solving sequence as a template for teaching. First the problem, then a tentative diagnosis, then a step to test the diagnosis, then the altered problem and a revised diagnosis. And on and on as teacher and student reason their way toward a diagnosis or plan of management.

My friend varied the routine with some patients, especially those who had been admitted recently. Here, he would ask the intern to present the history, physical findings, and routine laboratory data. When the intern finished, my friend would turn to the patient and check important points in the history and the examination himself. But he would then go back to the "What, in your opinion" questions.

I should add that he never mentioned the suspected diagnosis when we were in the presence of the patient. As he and the clerk or intern closed in on the identity of the disease, he would stop asking questions, turn to the patient, and summarize in simple words all the things we'd said. If the patient had questions, he would answer them. Then we would tell the patient good-bye and go into the hallway, where my friend would sum things up for us. I noticed that he avoided going to a conference room except to look at x-rays, and even there we remained standing—no one sat or leaned against a wall.

At one point, a resident cited a paper in the latest *New England Journal of Medicine*. My friend listened, then asked, "How does this information bear on our patient?" The question made it clear that every piece of our discussion had to be focused on the patient we were considering—on *this* patient in *this* bed.

From time to time, my friend would ask about chemistry and physiology, but these questions, too, were related to the patient. And again, he phrased most of the questions as if he were asking for opinions—"Thinking back to physiology, how could we explain . . . ?"

From that day onward, I picked up bits and pieces of information about teaching every time I ran into my friend or talked to people who had gone on rounds with him. But rather than report these fragments in the haphazard way they came to me, I'm going to present them as a conversation my friend and I might have had if we had gone to the lunch room after rounds and I had asked him questions over a cup of coffee. The conversation is, therefore, fictional, but its parts, insofar as I can trust my memory, are real.

"Do you find bedside teaching easy?"

"No. It's the hardest kind."

"Have you always taught this way?"

"No. It took a long time to settle on the format I use now. That it would take a long time would be expected, because learning to teach is a lifelong process, one that never ends."

"How did you hit on the routine you use?"

"It occurred to me that thinking about a patient means synthesizing information. Asking about the next step forces students and interns to do this, because if the step is always connected to what has gone before, synthesis is likely to follow. I am not, incidentally, after a diagnosis as much as I'm after the best next step, and why the young person chooses that step in preference to others. Often, as you know, the best next step is something simple, like calling the hospital where the patient had an x-ray a year earlier."

"I notice you often ask for opinions."

"Do I? Let's see, I suppose I do. But I don't do it consciously. What I try to do is stick to questions that make people think, questions that begin with 'why' or 'how' or 'in what way.' And come to think of it, I often ask, 'What, in your opinion, . . . ?' So you're right, I guess. The questions I ask are more likely to bring forth opinions than facts."

"What advice would you give a young doctor who wants to become a good clinical teacher?"

Speaking slowly, and pausing between the bits of advice, he replied, "Follow Osler's example and stay at the bedside, . . . listen to the patient, . . . stress the overwhelming importance of a careful history, . . . and practice, practice, practice."

My friend died a few years ago. I miss seeing him and having a chance to talk with him. Of the dozens of teachers I've gotten to know during my years in medicine, he is at the very top of my list.

## 25

## Making Diagnoses: The Early
## and Late Pathways

Telling students how physicians make diagnoses was easy when I was in medical school, forty years ago. It was easy because little was known about the diagnostic process or about the way physicians think. The only information given us came from Chester Keefer, chair of our department of medicine. "To become a good diagnostician," Dr. Keefer told us, "you must learn to think like Sherlock Holmes." So we took the steps we thought Holmes would have taken if he had been a physician. We searched for clues in the most detectivelike manner possible. Then we tried to diagnose the disease.

Now we know more about diagnosis-making, thanks to scientists who have studied the diagnostic process. We have learned, among other things, that physicians don't always follow the "search-diagnosis" sequence. Instead, they make a diagnosis early, then launch their search for clues.

To take a look at these switched-around steps and to see how they fit with those in other pathways, I shall briefly review the work of Aristotle, Francis Bacon, and Karl Popper, three philosophers who studied the way all of us reason and solve problems. Then I shall talk about a principle hidden in the early-diagnosis pathway, a principle so important it should be taught to students at the earliest possible time.

Aristotle, a great logician, gave us the syllogism, a pattern of reasoning with three parts—a major premise, a minor premise, and a conclusion. For example: (1) All ancient poets were dreamers (major premise), (2) Sappho was an ancient poet (minor premise), therefore, (3) Sappho was a dreamer (conclusion). With this, as with all syllogisms, the truth of the conclusion depends on the truth of the premises. If even one ancient poet was not a dreamer, our conclusion about Sappho may be wrong.

Despite such limitations, the syllogism was a dominant way of thinking from the time of Aristotle to the dawn of the Renaissance. In those days, people preferred to reason from old, accepted premises, rather than from fresh ideas. Fresh ideas—-especially fresh ideas about the Church or universe—could be dangerous. Galileo learned this when he defied the Church and agreed with Copernicus that the earth and planets revolved around the sun. Galileo was tried, forced to recant this belief, and imprisoned in his home. And Servetus, the man who said blood and air interact in the lungs, was doomed the moment he published his doubts about the Trinity in his small book, *Christianismi Restitutio*. He was seized, accused of heresy, and burned at the stake.

The syllogism survived and evolved into a classic thought pathway. We call it deduction.

A second pathway, a reaction to deduction, came from Francis Bacon, the English essayist and philosopher. Bacon lived four hundred years ago, during the reign of Elizabeth I. She ruled and Bacon worked in an era of glory and violence. Shakespeare wrote plays, the Royal Navy crushed the Spanish Armada, and Mary Stuart, Queen of Scots, lost her head on the executioner's block.

In the midst of these tumultuous times, Bacon took a risky step: he declared that the key to progress lay in recognizing the importance of science. The step was risky because it was, after all, common knowledge that scientists refused to confine their thinking to the guidelines of the Church. Then Bacon took a second risk. This time he said that deduction, the gift from the great Aristotle, was an inappropriate way for scientists to think. It was inappropriate, Bacon argued, because deduction assisted in "confirming and rendering inveterate the errors based on vulgar notions"rather than "searching after truth" (Adler and Wolff 1960, 138–39).

So Bacon proposed a different way of thinking, a way that started with observations, rather than premises. And once a series of observations had been made, the scientist looked for a theory that explained them. Bacon's method came to be known as induction ("to lead into") because the observations led the scientist into the explanation.

It was, I suppose, induction, or something like it, that we tried to use when we were medical students. We made observations while we took the history, examined the patient, and reviewed the laboratory data. Then, we put all the observations together and tried to name the disease.

Few of us knew that philosophers had questioned whether scientists actually use induction. We didn't know, for instance, about the skepticism of David Hume and C. S. Peirce or that of Karl Popper. Popper doubted that the mind would wait until all the observations had been made to come up with an explanation for them. Instead, Popper said, an explanation often suggests itself as soon as the mind grasps the problem (Magee, 50). We see this phenomenon in ourselves whenever we feel pain. If, for example, we wake up with an aching back, we instantly think, "I shouldn't have lifted the sofa yesterday." Or if we feel a twinge when ice water hits a tooth, we say, "I'll bet I have a cavity." Explaining the pain the second we feel it is as much a reflex as jerking our hand off a hot stove.

This, Popper said, is what scientists do. They often grasp the problem and think of a possible solution at almost the same time. So this pathway starts with the problem and a tentative solution. It then continues with steps that test whether the solution is sound.

Popper was talking about nonmedical scientists, but several studies have shown that seasoned physicians, too, think this way. When, for instance, Arthur Elstein and his colleagues asked experienced physicians to view films of the first few minutes of a physician's encounter with a person trained to simulate a patient, "nearly all [the physicians] began to generate diagnostic hypotheses within the earliest minutes of the encounter" (Elstein, Shulman, and Sprafka, 168).

Using a different protocol, Kassirer and Gorry found much the same thing. They had physicians think out loud as they met and questioned a man trained to play the role of a patient. The results showed "that specific diagnostic hypotheses were generated often with little more information than presenting complaints" (1978, 245).

In both studies physicians made diagnoses early, then continually refined the diagnoses as they carried out their search for clues. And in doing this, the physicians used the early-diagnosis pathway, the one with the switched-around steps. Yet, the view that a scientist or physician follows an inductive process—makes observations first, then looks for an explanation for them—continues to hold young doctors and many of their teachers in a grip of steel. "The belief that science proceeds from observation to theory," Popper said, "is still so widely and so firmly held that my denial of it is often met with incredulity. . . . But in fact the belief that we can start with pure observations alone, without any nature of a theory, is absurd" (Magee, 26).

Would it have helped for us to know about the early-diagnosis pathway when we were students? Yes. For hidden in the pathway is a principle of singular importance: physicians must look *for* things, not just look. They must feel, tap, and listen *for* things, not just feel, tap, and listen. Having a diagnosis in mind before they examine a patient impels doctors to do this. When, for example, they place a stethoscope over the heart, they go down a mental checklist of the abnormal sounds the heart might make if their tentative diagnosis is correct. Then they listen for the sounds, one at a time. Proctor Harvey, professor of medicine at Georgetown University, has for many years stressed the importance of this approach.

But what happens if doctors just look, feel, tap, and listen, rather than doing these things with a target in mind? They will miss clues. "Observation is always selective," Popper wrote, "It needs a chosen object, a definite task . . . a problem" (Magee, 26).

For all these reasons, students should be introduced to the early-diagnosis pathway—and to the principle of looking, feeling, tapping, and listening *for* things—as soon as their experience with patients enables them to use it. But this, in my experience, is seldom done.

We can't expect students to use the early-diagnosis pathway when they first start seeing patients, because they know little about signs and symptoms and even less about disease. So we start students with another pathway, a path in which they question and examine the patient before they try to name the illness. Hence, in this second pathway, the diagnosis comes late.

Students are introduced to the late-pathway in the all-important first-year course in physical diagnosis. Here, they learn to take a history by going down a long list of questions. The list is exhaustive and exhausting.It covers everything. They then examine the patient following another list, a list of things to look for, feel for, tap for, and listen for. This list, too, is all inclusive. Getting through this list, like getting through the list of questions, becomes an end in itself.

Students are warned against shortcuts, against any impulse that would cause them to depart from the lists. Sticking to the lists, their teachers tell them, ensures thoroughness, and thoroughness is a hallmark of a good physician.

They are also told that they must be "objective," which means, I suppose, that they should make observations in unbiased fashion, without any preconception of what the observations mean. This, of course, is nonsense. The very fact that an instructor tells a student to listen at the base of the heart suggests that the student may pick up useful information there.

The lists are inarguably important, yet they impose a handicap: they stifle spontaneous thought. Students are afraid to think aside, to come up with tentative diagnoses as they go along. They don't dare think independently until they've gotten through the lists.

But when students finish the course in physical diagnosis and move into the clerkships, most begin to think outside the lists. They get glimpses of other ways of thinking by watching attending physicians who have learned to use multiple thought pathways. The students then begin to use multiple paths themselves—-with timidity at first, and then with growing confidence.

Some students, however, stick to the lists. And so do some interns and residents. I learned this when I helped examine P and S residents who wanted to write the Boards in Internal Medicine. In each examination, I watched a senior resident question and examine a patient whom the resident hadn't seen before. I knew the residents well from having made teaching rounds with them. I also knew which residents the faculty considered top-notch and which they viewed as good but not quite tops. After examining residents in each of three years, I had found only one trait that seemed to separate the outstanding residents from the others: a willingness to depart temporarily from the lists. The excellent residents did this when they stumbled onto a clue that suggested an additional diagnosis. They would immediately pursue the clue, asking questions about it. Then, having finished, they would go back to working their way down the lists.

There was, for instance, M.P., a resident whom faculty members often said was as good as any resident they'd seen. I watched M.P. question a middle-aged man who'd come into the hospital with probable gall bladder disease. When M.P. asked the man about the jobs he'd held, the man mentioned working in the Brooklyn Navy Yard during World War II. The resident glanced up. The following exchange ensued:

"What did you do there?"

"Helped repair ships."

"Ever work below decks?"

"Sure."

"Any dust in the air?"

"Plenty."

"Ever strip asbestos off pipes?"

"Many times."

Then M.P. asked about breathlessness, cough, abnormal chest x-rays, and other things that go along with asbestosis. After adding the information to his notes, M.P. returned to the list of questions at the point where he'd left it when the patient mentioned working on ships.

The not-so-excellent residents came up with as many clues to diseases as the excellent residents, but the former would simply write down the clue, then continue through the list.

These observations raise a question: Should students be introduced to other thought paths, especially the early-diagnosis pathway,
in the same formal way they're taught the lists? Jerome Kassirer,
in an eloquent essay in the *New England Journal of Medicine* (1983),
answered the question with a resounding yes. Paul Cutler gave the
same answer in his book, *Problem Solving in Clinical Medicine: From
Data to Diagnosis* (1979).

> Students should be trained to form diagnostic hypotheses early so
> that their performance will more closely resemble that of the expert
> physician. These hypotheses are often generated during history taking
> and the student should branch into appropriate questions, look for
> confirmatory physical signs, and select diagnostic methods for testing
> or refuting [those] tentative impressions.
>
> Traditionally, students have been taught to gather a data base and
> solve a problem in separate inviolate orderly blocks. First, do a com-
> plete history. Second, do a complete physical examination. Then or-
> der routine laboratory tests, x-ray and ECG. When these are com-
> pleted, pick out the important clues from each of the three sources,
> then put them together so they fit a known diagnostic pattern as
> closely as possible. But this is not usually the way it's done "in real
> life" by practicing physicians. In fact, the teacher who sees patients
> does not do as he teaches. He begins to solve problems with his first
> question. (4)

To see if others share the view held by Kassirer and Cutler, I
searched eight textbooks on physical diagnosis for information about
pathways other than the lists. Only three books mentioned other
paths, and in these the comments were sparse. But I found an excellent discussion of diagnostic pathways in *The Principles and Practice of
Medicine* in a chapter written by Richard Johns, Nicholas Fortuin,
and Paul Wheeler (1988).

Now, to look at the combined use of the early and late paths and to
see how each serves us. The early-diagnosis path encourages synthe-

sis; the late-diagnosis path does not. The early path aids in problem solving; the late path may or may not help. The late path ensures thoroughness; the early path isn't thorough at all. The two pathways complement each other. They're like parts of a single whole. From what I've said, it's obvious that I agree with Kassirer and Cutler: the early-diagnosis pathway, as well as the late-diagnosis pathway, should be taught to students in a formal way.

## 26
## Two Other Uses of the Early and Late Pathways, One Bad and One Good

I have been speaking as if physicians used only two thought pathways. This, of course, is wrong. Physicians use all sorts of pathways: in *Problem Solving in Clinical Medicine*, Cutler listed thirteen types (38). I've also implied that physicians stick to one path when thinking about a patient. This, too, is wrong. The thoughts of physicians flit from path to path, just as everybody's thoughts jump around. But, since studies show that physicians often use the early-diagnosis pathway and we know they use the lists, I'm going to discuss two other ways we use the pathways, one bad and one good.

A regretable use of the late path arose in the following way. Instructors pound the lists into students with such force that even after students finish medical school and move through their internship and residency, they continue to give thoroughness priority, a practice that, on the whole, is laudable. But it stops being laudable when young physicians use the lists as a format for oral presentations. And young physicians everywhere do this. They fear they will be criticized if, in presenting a patient, they leave out one detail. Hence, a typical intern or resident starts a presentation with the chief complaint and, fifteen plodding minutes later, ends it with the diagnosis. No one—no student, intern, resident, or practicing physician—should present this way. The lists are perfect for the written record but totally unsuitable for an oral presentation. Listeners get lost in the flood of details.

George Sarton, the famed medical historian at Harvard, spoke to the difference between oral and written reports when he gave the Logan Clendening Lecture at the University of Kansas (1954). The oral presentation, Sarton said, should sketch the horizon; the written presentation should stick in the trees (1).

One way to sketch the horizon in an oral presentation is to use a journalistic approach. This means the presenter should:

1. Start with the most important feature of the illness, the suspected diagnosis. For example, "This thirty-year-old mother of three came to the hospital after a week of fever and sore throat. She has a few cells in her blood that look like blasts. We're afraid she has leukemia."
2. Pick out the points in the story relevant to the diagnosis, then present these and nothing else.
3. Remember that any patient, no matter how complicated, can be presented in five minutes, and most in three.

Young physicians will be wary of starting with the diagnosis, because everyone knows the diagnosis comes last. Saving it for last is a throwback to the time when there was little effective treatment for anything, and the diagnosis was all. Hence, the presenter, like an actor speaking lines, kept the dramatic flourish till the end. Nowadays, the best ending is to give the next step the presenter plans to take. In the story of the woman with the suspected leukemia, for instance, the presenter could end with, "We shall look at the bone marrow this morning."

Presentations should be models of synthesis and brevity. And if, at the end, the listeners ask questions, the presenter should be pleased. For questions mean the listeners have understood well enough to ask about details.

A good use of the early-diagnosis path is helping us to follow a student's thinking when he or she is analyzing a patient's problem. The path also shows us the weak points in the tools we're now using, tools like the process called patient-management problem (PMP).

The PMP asks about next steps: "You would then order . . . ?" "You would next perform . . . ?" or you would take this step or that? The PMP also provides information on the patient's condition: "The woman remained breathless, so . . . " But the PMP does not tell us how these bits of information influence the test-taker's thoughts about a diagnosis. A comparison with Karl Popper's problem-solving sequence shows the steps that the PMP omits.

| *Popper's Sequence* | *The PMP* |
| --- | --- |
| Problem | "This eighty-year-old . . ." |
| Tentative Dx | _____ |
| Error-correcting step | "You would order . . . ?" |
| Altered problem | "The test you ordered is negative." |
| Refined Dx | _____ |
| Error-correcting step | "You would next . . . ?" |
| Altered problem | "The patient continues . . ." |
| Refined Dx | _____ |

The comparison provides a blueprint of the gaps that new testing tools should fill. In the meantime, alternatives to the PMP include discussions at the bedside, where the teacher, through skillful use of "What," "Why," and "In what way" questions, can follow the entire problem-solving sequence. Essay questions, too, can do this, but multiple-choice questions cannot. Multiple choice questions test a student's fund of facts and ability to recall the facts.

Little else.

## 27
## Are We Socratic Teachers?

As the years have gone by and I've listened to discussions of clinical teaching, I've come to believe that many of us view ourselves as disciples of Socrates. Colleagues have told me they rely heavily on the Socratic method, especially when teaching at the bedside or in small, informal groups. Some have said that Socratic teaching is the very heart of clinical instruction, that clinical medicine could not, in all probability, be taught in any other way. When I've asked, "How would you describe the Socratic method?" the answers have had a sameness about them. Most colleagues have said that the method consists of teaching by asking questions.

Socrates did ask lots of questions. But do the words "to teach by asking questions" adequately describe the method that brought him fame? If teachers simply ask their students questions, can teachers claim mastery of the Socratic technique?

To look into the matter, I shall go back to the dialogue in *Meno* where Socrates shows the young slave how to reason about geometry. I shall review the background of the dialogue, look at the questions Socrates asks, and examine the way he asks them. Then we can try to decide whether we teach like Socrates taught.

We are in Greece, in the fifth century B.C., at the time when Socrates could usually be found in the marketplace, gathering young people around him, urging them to define their terms. On this day, Socrates and Meno are talking about virtue and the way virtue may be defined. As they debate whether virtue is innate or learned, they begin to discuss the mechanics of learning and the role the teacher plays.

An earlier version of section 27 appeared in *Transactions of the American Clinical and Climatological Association* 90 (1978): 109–15.

Meno, a sophist—and, therefore, a professional educator—seems to believe that a good teacher provides students with useful information (Brumbaugh 1962, 57–58). Socrates disagrees, arguing that a student can learn only things the student already knows, so the duty of the teacher is to help the student recollect the buried bits and pieces then fit them into new forms. Curious and skeptical, Meno challenges Socrates to demonstrate the process. Socrates chooses for his demonstration a problem in geometry.

The problem is this: Given a square with sides of known length, how long will the sides of a second square be if the area of the second square is twice that of the first? The answer is that the side of the second square will equal the length of the diagonal of the first square. To reach this answer, a student needs to be able to compare areas of squares with areas of triangles. Hence, the problem Socrates chooses is difficult and complicated.

Socrates needs a subject for the demonstration and asks Meno to provide one. Meno turns to a group of attendants standing nearby and beckons to a young slave. As the boy steps forward, Socrates asks one of the dramatic questions in the annals of education: "He is Greek, and speaks Greek, does he not?" Instead of inquiring about the boy's knowledge of geometry or his ability to reason, Socrates simply wants assurance that he and the boy speak the same tongue.

When Meno provides the assurance, Socrates scratches a square in the sand beside their feet and divides it into four smaller squares by drawing lines connecting the midpoints of opposite sides. Then with Socrates and the boy in the center, and the others gathered around, the dialogue begins.

> "Tell me, boy, do you know a figure like this is a square?"
> "I do."
> "And you know that a square has its four sides equal?"
> "Certainly."
> "And these lines I've drawn through the square are also equal?"
> "Yes."

"A square may be of any size?"
"Certainly." (Jowett 1937, 361)

These questions, typical of those in the rest of the dialogue, are simple, clear, and easily answerable. They have a disarming informality, a conversational tone. But when we look at the questions closely, we find their simplicity is deceptive. Far from being random and unstructured, the questions have features that can be readily identified.

The first and most important feature is that each of the questions calls for a judgment or an opinion, then a yes-or-no answer. Further, if we analyze all fifty-two questions in the dialogue, we find that more than half are this same type.

Socrates plainly tells us that opinions are the secret of his method. Part-way through the dialogue he turns to Meno and says, "Do you watch and see if you find me telling or explaining anything to him, instead of eliciting his opinion." And by soliciting one opinion after another, Socrates leads the boy toward a sharply defined goal—the length of the side of the second square.

A second feature of the questions is that Socrates seldom asks for facts (Klein 1965, 103). And when he does ask for a fact, it is of the simplest sort—"How many are twice two feet?"

The reason Socrates stays away from facts seems clear. His goal is to get the boy to reason, and to do this, he needs to keep the conversation moving. The boy, like any student, gladly offers an opinion, no matter how difficult the question, so soliciting an opinion guarantees an answer. But asking for a fact is risky, because the boy may not know the fact. If this happens, the conversation falters and loses momentum, like a sailboat going into irons.

Is it possible to teach medicine by avoiding facts and asking for opinions? J. Willis Hurst has said it is. In his instructive book, *Notes from a Chairman* (1987), Hurst set forth his thoughts on teaching and suggested an approach Socrates would have admired. Instead of asking a student to name a half dozen causes of diastolic rumbles, for example, he recommends asking if the student can think of factors that might cause a rumble to develop. The two questions resemble each other, yet the difference between them is vast. The first tests the size of the student's fund of facts and the student's ability to recall the facts. The second tests the student's ability to think.

A third feature of Socratic questions is that each suggests its answer: each question leads the boy to the correct reply. So if we want to teach as Socrates taught the slave, we must ask leading questions, a type we are taught to avoid when talking with patients.

A fourth and last feature centers on the sequence of the questions. Seemingly random, the order has a formidable precision, equivalent to that of an algorithm with multiple binary points. The incremental increase in information needed to answer the next question is so small as to be almost imperceptible, yet the increase is essential to the series, a series so tightly structured that it has been called the first programmed text (Cohen 1962, 772).

Having considered the features of Socrates' questions, we turn to the way he asks them, how he talks to the boy. Socrates offers encouragement, "Very good: I like to hear what you think." At the same time, he builds the boy's confidence by phrasing the questions so the boy can answer almost every one of them: only once is the boy forced to say, "I do not know." Most important of all, Socrates creates the illusion that he and the boy are learning together, that they are equals working toward a common goal. Socrates makes the student the center of the exercise. He lets the student star.

Repeatedly, through the ages, the dialogue in *Meno* has been held up as the supreme example of the teaching art. Yet, it is not this dialogue we think of when we hear the Socratic method mentioned. Medical students might be surprised to hear that their Socratic professors offer encouragement, ask only answerable questions, and pose as equals working toward a common goal.

And whether or not medical students would be surprised, law students would almost certainly be. Evidence for this comes from the delightful book *ONE-L* (1977), by Scott Turow. The book is an account of Turow's experience as a first-year student at the Harvard Law School. Early in the book, Turow characterizes student reaction to Socratic teaching in these paragraphs:

> In a way I'm looking forward to Socratic instruction. I've heard so much about it since I applied to law school—it will at least be interesting to see what it's like.
>
> The general run of student reaction is most succinctly expressed in a comment I heard from David this summer, the day he showed me around the law school.... "This is Langdell Hall," he said, " . . . named for the late Christopher Columbus Langdell, who was dean of Harvard Law School in the late nineteenth century. Dean Langdell is best known as the inventor of the Socratic method."
>
> David lowered his hand and looked sincerely at the building. "May he rot in hell," David said. (40)

Those who've read the book know why David wished this fate on the departed dean. Professors of law, like professors of medicine, often bombard their students with questions, push their students steadily backward, keep the students on uncertain ground. In doing this, the professors use another type of Socratic questioning, a procedure resembling cross-examination. It is the approach Socrates uses when talking to Meno, when speaking to us, his audience, when dealing with people his own size.

Socrates was always teaching, so most of his conversations embodied a student-teacher relationship. Yet, only in *Meno* do we have a chance to watch Socrates talk both to a senior person and to a boy who is a student in the traditional sense. Only in *Meno* do we have a chance to see the two approaches laid out side by side.

Both approaches are effective, but they are very different, so the use of one or the other must be a deliberate choice. With either, the teacher acts as a midwife, by helping the student mobilize information, a role Socrates continually plays (Farrar 1977).

The approach espoused by Dean Langdell has many positive features, yet it also has the drawback Turow mentions when summarizing his personal view:

> That night in May, the faculty panel roundly agreed to the continuing vitality of the Socratic method. I would not differ directly, but the peculiar privilege which Socraticism grants a teacher to invade the security of every student in the room means that in the wrong hands it can become an instrument of terror. I never felt that my education gained by my being frightened, and I was often scared in class. Law faculties have too long excused, in the name of academic freedom, a failure to hold colleagues within basic bounds of decency. (296)

The potential for abuse is constantly with us. It exists for professors of medicine, just as it exists for professors of law.

In light of the foregoing, physicians can, it seems to me, say they teach like Socrates taught the slave if they

ignore the background of the student,
ask for opinions,
avoid facts,
have a clearly defined goal, and
let the student star.

Montaigne admired these principles, just as he admired Socrates, and he expressed his admiration in this way: "Our tutors never stop bawling into our ears, as though they were pouring water into a funnel; and our task is only to repeat what has been told us. . . . I don't want [the teacher] to think and talk alone, I want him to listen to his pupil speaking in his turn. Socrates, and later Arcesilaus, first had their disciples speak, and then they spoke to them" (110).

Then Montaigne ends by quoting Cicero: "Obest plerumque iis qui discere volunt, auctoritas eorum qui docent"—"Sometimes, the authority of the teacher gets in the way of those who wish to learn."

## 28
## Four Comments on
## Medical Training

### Comment 1

The simplest way to improve a lecture course for medical students is to let one person give all the talks. The second best way is to divide the course into big parts—say, three—then let one lecturer give each part.

These suggestions will bring cries of anguish from faculty members who believe medical students should be taught by a parade of specialists. These faculty members may be right, but my hunch is that, at the student level, the benefit of being taught by specialists is small compared to the inestimable value of continuity. A student needs to be able to ask the teacher the day after the lecture about things the student didn't understand. In medical schools, in many courses, the teacher who lectured isn't there the next day.

Critics will argue that giving all the lectures in a course is a back-breaking task for one person. That's true. They will also argue that others in the department will want to lecture. That's true too. But faculty members might spread the burden around by having different members teach the course in different years.

### Comment 2

Insofar as interns and residents are concerned, the popularity of a clinician as a consultant is determined, to a considerable extent, by the proximity of the clinician to where the interns and residents work. If a faculty member walks around the patient-care units at odd hours, house officers will ask his or her opinion. Interns and residents are unbelievably busy, chronically behind on things they are supposed to do. Hence, they feel that they can't spare time to go look for a consultant: they'll consult the physician who comes near them.

So when I hear attending physicians complain that house officers don't consult them, I know the reason: those physicians aren't walking around the units.

## Comment 3

No physician should take advice on clinical teaching from anyone who is not better known for something else. The great clinical teachers have made their reputations in research, clinical care, or writing—not education.

## Comment 4

A chair should never hire physicians who say they teach because they wish to help the young. Clinicians teach for the ego boost it gives them and for the satisfaction that comes from doing a hard job well.

Altruism may, on occasion, play a role. When it does, the role is small.

## 29
## Training the Good Generalist

Fifteen or so years ago, at a meeting of the Association of Professors of Medicine, I listened to a discussion of the ratio of generalists to subspecialists, a topic that had received sporadic attention at earlier meetings of the group. On this day, however, the ratio had acquired a new importance—indeed, an urgency—because a large manpower study had revealed that the existing ratio of two generalists to one subspecialist would, if current trends continued, be reversed during the following two decades.

This prospect was, to say the least, alarming. After all, senators, congressional representatives, and a variety of health planners had told us that our great need was for physicians who practice general medicine, physicians who, in the eyes of the government and public, are the exact opposite of those trained in subspecialties.

Then, too, the AMA's *Report of the Citizen's Commission on Graduate Medical Education* (1966) had declared, "The rise in specialization has been accompanied by an alarming decline in the number of physicians who devote themselves to continuing and comprehensive care of the whole individual." So, at our meeting that morning, we talked about ways to increase the number of generalists. And as suggestions were put forward, then debated and assessed, two ideas received particular attention.

The first was to limit the number of residents entering subspecialty training. This step, an obvious one, would not only protect the existing two-to-one ratio but also eventually improve it, since the number of residents was growing yearly and the extra residents, if denied subspecialty training, would presumably stay in general medicine. But several people worried that the FTC would torpedo any

An earlier version of section 29 appeared as an editorial in *The Pharos* (Alpha Omega Alpha Honor Medical Society) Spring 1980, 32.

constraint that interfered with a young person's freedom of choice. And since no one could rule out this possibility, we set the first idea aside.

The second idea was to expand the programs designed to train "broad-based generalists." The logic here was inarguably compelling. What better way to produce generalists than to give residents extra training in general medicine?

Yet, as I looked around the room and identified friends I knew to be good generalists, I realized that each had trained in a subspecialty. None, so far as I knew, had written a subspecialty examination, but each had had enough subspecialty training to be identified with a subspecialty field.

Struck by the observation, then concerned that the phenomenon might be peculiar to chairs, I began writing down the names of the best generalists I'd known during my years in medicine. At the end of an hour, I had listed two dozen people, people with credentials as different as their personalities. Some had been chairs of departments, some had been academicians but not chairs, and some had not been connected with medical schools. Three-quarters, however, were linked to subspecialties.

The list raised a puzzling question: does training in a subspecialty strengthen the possibility that a young physician will become a good generalist? At the time, I couldn't answer the question, but now I've come to believe the answer might be yes.

Once immersed in a strong subspecialty program, trainees learn to be critical—of the literature, of patient care, of new drugs and interventions. They develop a respect for the fallibility of measuring instruments and learn that the numbers they provide can as easily mislead as help. They learn that framing a sharp question is the essential first step in solving a problem, whether the problem arises at the bedside or in the laboratory. Most important of all, trainees will acquire perspective about the practice of medicine: by learning one subspecialty in depth, they become able to gauge the limits of their knowledge in other areas and know when to call for help.

In 1980 John G. Kemeny, then president of Dartmouth College, touched on this subject in a colloquium that addressed the question, "What does it take to be an educated person in today's world?" Breadth of education, Kemeny said, continues to be the first consideration. But he then added, "I'm a great believer in the value of the major, and it almost doesn't matter what you major in. Taking some subject and going into it in great depth—as intellectual discipline—that's absolutely essential."

How long would an aspiring generalist have to train in a subspecialty to achieve these benefits? One year would probably be enough. Suggesting a single year for any purpose, however, has been to invite a storm of protests. One objection has been that the year would produce a dilettante, a hobbyist, a demispecialist. Another has been that one year would be difficult to fund. Still another has been that most trainees would succumb to temptation and end up limiting their practice to the subspecialty.

This last argument has more scare appeal than practical importance, for becoming a generalist involves—if nothing else—a conscious decision to try to embrace all of medicine. Having made the decision, young physicians will likely maintain their broad interests, whether or not they train in a subspecialty. And they will spend their lives trying "to understand the whole of knowledge, as well as one man can" (Van Doren 1959, 14).

So, one way to train a good generalist, a generalist another physician will go to or send family members to or refer friends to, is to expose a young doctor to intense training in a subspecialty.

Since 1980, when I first published these thoughts, the training of general physicians has assumed even greater importance, because health maintenance agencies have opted to sign up generalists, rather than higher-priced subspecialists, to care for their patients. In light of this new emphasis on general medicine, would a year of subspecialty training still be a good idea?

Yes, especially for generalists who plan to enter academic medicine. These generalists will want to work toward tenure, and their path will be smoothed if they are able to do research. An exposure to a subspecialty would enable them to initiate research projects or collaborate in on-going projects in their subspecialty. When faculty members have done this, it partly relieves one of a chair's headaches: how to get tenure for clinical people.

## *30*
## Why a Wise Chair Emulates Great Leaders, and What Great Leaders Teach

Machiavelli knew the importance of emulating great leaders, and he underscored this importance in the following way: "For as men almost always follow the beaten track of others, and proceed in their actions by imitation, . . . so a wise man should ever follow the ways of great men. . . . Even if his merits do not quite equal theirs, yet they may in some measure reflect their greatness. He should do as the skillful archer, who, seeing that the object he desires to hit is too distant . . . aims higher than the destined mark, not for the purpose of sending his arrow to that height, but so that by this elevation it may reach the desired aim" (20).

With these thoughts in mind, let us examine the lives of three physicians who headed medical units in the middle of this century and who, by any yardstick, were great leaders in their fields. We shall look at their traits and habits and at the qualities they had in common. Then we shall see what they taught the young men and women who came to them for training.

An earlier version of section 30 appeared in *The Pharos* (Alpha Omega Alpha Honor Medical Society), ⟨issue, date, pages to come⟩.

### Chester Keefer

Chester Keefer was chair of medicine at Boston University. Five feet ten, with square jaw and authoritarian bearing, he quizzed students publicly and intensively and, some would say, mercilessly. But he treated interns, residents, and faculty members the same way. Everyone, at some time or other, got grilled by The Professor, as if he kept a check list in his pocket and made sure each person got raked over from time to time.

There was, for instance, the July morning in 1949 when Keefer was going to make chief-of-service rounds with the head nurse, his brand new house staff, and a half-dozen of us third-year clerks. By five minutes of ten, we were standing in the foyer of the teaching service, uniforms starched and spotless, eyes riveted on the clocklike indicator above the elevator door.

On the stroke of the hour, the indicator turned to our floor and stopped, the door slid open, and Keefer and the chief resident stepped out. Glaring at the floor, Keefer swiveled to his left, marched down the hall, and turned into the room of Mr. M., a seventy-year-old man who'd had a heart attack. The rest of us hurried after Keefer, crowded into the room behind him, grouped ourselves around the bed.

Keefer snapped, "Whose case is this?" The intern stepped forward and presented the patient. He gave the history, told what he'd found on physical examination, and summarized the results of the laboratory tests. When he'd finished, there was silence. Then Keefer turned to the chief resident and growled, "Now, who really knows this case?"

Balanced against this fierce approach was the fact that Keefer gave his students and staff top priority. His responsibility for their training was his number one concern. This was surprising, because much of his time was taken up by special assignments—things like supervising the distribution of penicillin after World War II and serving as special assistant to the Secretary of Health. Yet he seldom missed his Monday rounds with house officers and clerks. And his rounds were—to say the least—spectacular, because Keefer was a superb clinician, a man who had spent endless hours at the bedside. His broad experience, prodigious memory, and knowledge of disciplines other than medicine made his rounds legendary.

Keefer's Germanic system suited many people perfectly: they liked the idea of knowing exactly what they could and could not do. And anyone willing to meet Keefer's high standards could count on his friendship. For despite his steely manner, he looked out for his people. He'd do anything to get them to the places they wanted to go.

## André Cournand

André Cournand was head of the Cardio-Pulmonary Laboratory at Bellevue Hospital in New York. A broad-shouldered man of average height, Cournand had the graceful movements of an athlete. Even in middle life, he was lithe and muscular, with a carriage that reflected boyhood hours spent on soccer and football fields.

Born in France and educated at the University of Paris, Cournand was every inch a scholar. He knew the humanities as well as he knew science and, on a typical morning, would talk with excitement about the book that had kept him up until all hours—one by Goethe, by Voltaire, or by Poincaré. In talking about his reading, as in all his activities, Cournand radiated enthusiasm. He had the "god within" that Pasteur prized and talked about (Dubos 1986).

But when he lectured, Cournand could be incoherent. If he talked without a manuscript, he was disorganized; if he used a manuscript, he read at breakneck speed. Hints from friends went unheeded. Then, on a spring day in the late 1940s, the following events took place.

Cournand was to read a paper in the afternoon session of a meeting of physicians. Just before lunch, he sought out Kenneth Donald, one of the fellows in Cournand's laboratory, a man who would later be chair of medicine at Edinburgh. Their conversation, Ken told me, went like this: "Ken," Cournand said, "I've heard that some people have trouble understanding my talks. Have you heard this?" "If I ever did," said Donald, opting for tact rather than full disclosure, "it would have been only one or two." "It couldn't be my accent," Cournand continued. "Certainly not." "Some say I talk too fast. Is that possible?" "It's possible for any of us to talk too fast." "Then, Ken, I'd like you to sit in front of the podium when I read my paper, and if I go too fast, raise your hand."

So that afternoon, when Cournand stepped to the microphone in the packed auditorium, Ken Donald was in the seat directly in front of him. Cournand began slowly, but in a few moments, picked up speed. Donald raised his hand to shoulder level. Cournand accelerated, and Donald raised his hand to the level of his ear. When Cournand went still faster, Donald stuck his hand straight up. "By the end of the talk, Dr. Cournand was forgotten," Donald said later. "All eyes—except those of Dr. Cournand—were riveted on my hand."

But Cournand's troubles as a speaker were trivial compared to his many strengths. He was, for instance, eminently approachable. He also had the knack of making junior people feel that their work was important, that their studies just might bring a Nobel Prize. And Cournand was nothing if not a friend to his people. His overriding priority was the well-being of his staff.

## Dickinson W. Richards

The third leader was Dickinson W. Richards, director of the First (Columbia) Medical Service at Bellevue. Tall and spare and ramrod straight, he was self-contained and shy. Richards seldom spoke and, when he did, never used two words if one would do. Conny, his wife, once said to my wife and me, "Dick's in Chicago, and it's delightful.

He says much more in his cards and letters than he ever says at home."

Richards was every inch a scholar. He had mastered Greek and Latin, and these noble languages had become a part of him. It was as if he were in his third incarnation, having lived the first in Periclean Athens, the second in Augustan Rome.

At the bedside, Richards was warm, sympathetic, and interested, the sort of courtly physician patients love. But in the lecture hall, he—like Cournand—had trouble. Richards spoke about this in 1968 at a dinner honoring him just before retirement: "If ever a man had teaching thrust upon him, it was I. I didn't like it very well, and I couldn't manage it at all. Before an audience, any audience, I was embarrassed and flustered. If I failed to write my message down, I forgot it; if I did, I lost my place. The students, naturally, were as cold as any stone; snapped their seats up after the first few sentences, and walked out; eventually would look into the auditorium and not come in at all."

But when it came to writing, Richards had few equals. Anyone doubting this should read his presidential address to the Association of American Physicians (1962), especially the part about what it means to be a doctor (quotes from which can be found below, in section 38). Richards was equally formidable when it came to research. Here, he was the ultimate skeptic: data had to be convincing, or he was not impressed.

In the political arena, Richards was a dedicated liberal. In his quiet way, he warred against social injustice and apathetic public servants, using as weapons the essay and the letter to the editor. One such letter sparked a revolt that brought to its knees the Department of Health of New York City, an agency that had developed a callous disregard for patients and had let its hospitals lapse into decay.

Richards, like Keefer and Cournand, had a deep and abiding interest in the well-being of his people. They knew that if they gave the best they had within them, Richards would be their friend for life.

Keefer, Cournand, and Richards were very different, yet they shared two traits. One was a love of learning, the other an interest in their staffs.

But what, exactly, did the three teach the young men and women who flocked to them for training? Was it how to use digitalis, how to test data with statistics, how to drain water from a chest? None taught any of these things. Others taught the trainees everyday research and medicine. Keefer, Cournand, and Richards taught things that had no immediate practical use.

They taught things like humanity and decency and discipline. They let their young friends watch a leader work, up close and continually. They let them see a leader stumble and make mistakes. And fate, sad to say, forced each of the three, at one time or another, to let their young colleagues see how good people endure misfortune: the death of a friend, the loss of a wife.

Most teachers teach through lectures, conferences, or demonstrations. Great leaders teach by being what they are.

# 31
# Scientists and Criticism, Chairs and Criticism

Francis Bacon told us how he believed a scientist should work and think. The scientist should make observations, then devise a theory to explain them. If the theory stands up when others test it, we conclude that the theory is correct. We then add it to our store of knowledge as a principle or general law.

Two hundred years after Bacon, David Hume pondered the same subject and had trouble with Bacon's process. Hume was skeptical that observations or experiments, no matter how many or how significant, could prove beyond doubt that a theory was correct. He questioned whether an infinite number of observations protected a scientist from having the next observation contradict the law the scientist had discovered. The observation, for instance, that the moon changed from new to full this month, provides no assurance the moon will do the same thing in the months to come.

And two hundred years after Hume expressed skepticism, Karl Popper voiced similar doubts. Popper refused to believe that anything could be proved with certainty (Magee, 19–21). All knowledge is provisional, Popper said, and will remain permanently so. At no stage can we prove what we believe to be true, because it is always possible it will turn out to be false. Xenophanes had made similar comments twenty-four hundred years earlier. "As for certain truth, no man has known it" (36–37).

Then Popper had an insight that would bring him both fame and notoriety. The insight was that there is a logical asymmetry between proving something right and proving it wrong. The asymmetry is this: whereas no number of experiments can prove a theory right, one experiment can suggest that the theory is partly or wholly wrong. Which means, Popper said, that a scientific law can be conclusively falsified, even though it cannot be conclusively verified. This led Popper to suggest that science be defined as "that which can be falsified."

As might have been expected, Popper's definition drew fire from scientists. Some said the definition was nihilistic, that refusal to believe that anything could be proved undermined the scientific enterprise. If Popper's definition of science were adopted, they complained, scientists would hesitate to say anything at all. And Peter Medawar called attention to a practical difficulty: "Falsification is not itself immune to error" (1990, 21). The experiment that appears to falsify may be wrong.

Anticipating such objections, Popper said scientists could qualify their conclusions with a phrase like "to the best of our knowledge" (Magee, 19). Better, scientists could consider several theories, then justify their preference for one theory over the others.

Having put forward the principle of falsification, Popper discussed the consequences that automatically followed. The most important was that the goal of scientists should be to falsify hypotheses, both their own and those of others.

Magee (16–18) helps us understand this approach by telling about a fictional scientist who, while working at sea level, notices that water boils at 100 degrees centigrade. When additional measurements confirm the observation, the scientist publishes the results and suggests that water boiling at 100 degrees is a general law.

At this point, Magee, quoting Popper, says the scientist should quit looking for additional support for the law and search instead for exceptions to it. The scientist should search for information that would either falsify the law or show it to be only partly right. To this end, the scientist might, Magee says, repeat the experiment at an altitude. There, water would boil at a lower temperature, and when observations were made at other altitudes, an inverse linear relation between altitude and the boiling point would emerge. These new experiments would falsify the first theory, but at the same time, generalize and expand it.

One of the most important consequences of the idea of falsification is that scientists must be critics: they must continually criticize what they themselves and others have done. Popper believed that it is through criticism, and criticism alone, that knowledge grows (Magee, 6). In his book, *The Open Society and Its Enemies*, Popper criticized Plato and Marx. The arguments were compelling—they undermined the idea that communistic government in any form could be made to work. Yet, Popper paid a price for what he'd written: he became known as a man who criticized other people. This accusation was a bit off the point, because Popper criticized the ideas of Plato and Marx, not Plato and Marx themselves. But for some people, the slightest hint that a person is a critic evokes a feeling of distaste. Critics are second guessers, these people say. Somebody has to do something before a critic can criticize.

Not everyone feels this way, of course. Linda Winer, drama columnist for *Newsday*, offered a friendlier view of critics in her line of work (1992). She was, she said, "a sucker for opinions about the arts. I like it when there are lots of voices with lots of things to say about what happened in the theater last night—even when they make me nuts. I even like it when every critic seems to have been at an entirely different event, because it reminds audiences, not that critics are stupid, but that the arts, like life, are complicated." And so it is in science. Lots of voices saying different things keep science moving forward.

Popper, incidentally, was talking about nonmedical science. How about criticism in medical research? Should clinical investigators try to falsify theories published by their colleagues? And should clinical investigators welcome criticism as Popper says nonmedical scientists should?

I can answer the last question for myself and my colleagues when we were young and trying to build our reputations in research. Instead of welcoming criticism, we feared it. We stayed in a perpetual state of anxiety that someone would show our work was wrong. Looking back, I see that our fear stemmed mostly from vanity. But it also stemmed from the worry that a granting agency would be more impressed by work that had withstood attacks than by work that had been destroyed by them.

Our attitude created a dilemma, just as Popper said it would, for we found it was seldom possible to discover something without having subsequent work modify our understanding of what we'd discovered. Peter Harris, Simon Marks Professor Emeritus at the University of London, likened a beginning investigator to someone assigned the task of patting flat a small area of a large sheet of damp, wrinkled, tissue paper, laid out on the floor. When he gets the assigned area flat, he tries to extend his work by patting flat an area adjacent to the first. But doing so wrinkles the first, so he has to reach behind and pat the first area back in place. Eventually, Dr. Harris said, the person will be patting with both hands and feet, trying to reach out in new directions while trying to protect what has already been done.

Let's now consider whether a chair might profit from criticism in the way Popper says a scientist can. "Not only working scientists," Magee says, "can be liberated" by criticism.

> For all of us, in all our activities, the notions that we can do better only by finding out what can be improved and improving on it; and therefore that short-comings are to be actively sought out, not concealed or passed over; and that critical comment from others, far from being resented, is an invaluable aid to be insisted upon and welcomed, are liberating to a remarkable degree.
>
> It may be difficult to get people—conditioned to resent criticism and expect it to be resented, and therefore to keep silent about their own mistakes and others'—to provide the criticism on which improvement depends; but no one can possibly give us more service than by showing us what is wrong with what we think or do; and the bigger the fault, the bigger the improvement made possible by its revelation. The man who welcomes and acts on criticism will prize it almost above friendship: the man who fights it out of concern to maintain his position is clinging to non-growth. (32–33)

But no matter how useful the information, criticism hurts. James Harvey Robinson knew this and dealt with it in his small book *The Mind in the Making* (1921).

> We sometimes find ourselves changing our minds without any resistance or heavy emotion, but if we are told that we are wrong, we resent the imputation and harden our hearts. We are incredibly heedless in the formation of our beliefs, but find ourselves filled with an illicit passion for them when anyone proposes to rob us of their companionship. It is obviously not the ideas themselves that are dear to us, but our self-esteem, which is threatened. We are by nature stubbornly pledged to defend our own from attack, whether it be our person, our family, our property, or our opinion. (36)

So, criticism is hard to take. And for a chair, it carries a risk, because excessive criticism, especially excessive public criticism, can weaken a chair's control.

The way a chair deals with criticism must be a deliberate choice. One way is to encourage it, without setting limits on what the members of the department can say. Opting for this course will bring the benefits Magee talked about, but at the same time it will put the chair's security at risk.

The second option is a middle course, like the one Machiavelli suggested. "A prince," he said, "should always take counsel, but only when he wants it, and not when others wish to thrust it upon him; in fact, he should rather discourage persons from tendering him advice unsolicited by him" (106). Here, as with the first option, the chair invites criticism, but this time sets limits on it. In theory, this is a good approach, but in practice, it's often hard to hold people to pre-set limits. And, in fact, Machiavelli himself modified the approach, suggesting that a prince "be an extensive questioner, and a patient listener to the truth respecting the things inquired about, and should even show his anger in case anyone should, for some reason, not tell him the truth" (106).

The third method is to let the department know, in one way or another, that criticism isn't welcome. Chairs in the first half of this century often operated this way, but a present-day chair considering this option should first ponder a comment Popper made: "The wrong view of science betrays itself in the craving to be right" (Magee, 32). And it's just possible that the wrong view of leadership betrays itself the same way.

## 32

# The Importance of the Second Notebook

All interns carry a notebook in their pocket, a bent, bulging notebook crammed with hard-to-remember facts. Typical entries include normal levels of blood electrolytes, point systems for diagnosing diseases of unknown origin, and dosage schedules for little-used drugs. The notebook is an essential part of an intern's medical practice. It's a crutch, a security blanket, an everpresent source of help.

My chief, Chester Keefer, told us we should carry a second notebook, a notebook for questions, not for facts. "It's a good idea," Dr. Keefer said, "to spend a few minutes each day writing down questions that come up when you're seeing patients." Such questions would start us thinking about research, he said.

I accepted on faith every word Dr. Keefer uttered, yet I wondered whether medical researchers actually kept such notebooks. I hadn't seen a notebook with questions in it, but then I hadn't seen many medical researchers up close either. One day, more than ten years after I'd left Dr. Keefer's service, I saw such a notebook. I stumbled across it when I picked up a small monograph by Hoff, Guillemin, and Guillemin (1967) on the *Cahier Rouge*, the notebook with red covers found in Claude Bernard's effects four years after his death. The red notebook not only contained lots of questions but also let me see how a medical scientist thinks. And it introduced me to Claude Bernard, the man who, in the last century, laid the foundation for clinical research.

Before I speak about the notebook, I shall talk about Bernard himself. He was born in France, in the village of St. Julien, on 12 July 1813. His father was a teacher, his mother, a homemaker. He attended the village school and was, we're told, an undistinguished student. At the age of eighteen, he obtained a part-time job with a pharmacist, a job that would influence the course of his later life. One of his tasks was to deliver drugs to the local veterinary school, and Bernard found the school fascinating.

His great interest lay in the theater, however, and he wrote and produced several plays. He solicited the opinion of a Parisian professor and drama critic named Giardin. Doubting that Bernard would do well as a playwright and knowing about his work at the pharmacy, Giardin suggested that Bernard study medicine. And at the age of twenty, Bernard entered medical school in Paris.

In the course of his training, while serving as an intern at Hotel Dieu, Bernard was assigned to the clinical service of François Magendie, the famed physician and physiologist. Magendie, recognizing Bernard's talent, made him his laboratory assistant, and in short order Bernard left clinical medicine and embarked on a career in physiology. He wrote his first paper on the chorda tympani. Then he began a study of digestion that led to his doctoral thesis, *The Gastric Juice and Its Role in Nutrition.*

As he pursued his interest in the GI tract, Bernard noticed that fats, unlike other foodstuffs, were not digested in the stomach. They remained unchanged, he found, until they reached the duodenum and the mouth of the common duct. Then they were emulsified. So Bernard hit on the idea that the pancreas secretes a substance or substances that prepare fats for absorption. When he subsequently proved this was true, the work was hailed as a landmark achievement. Bernard was "the first scientist to appreciate the importance of internal glandular secretions" (Bender 1962, 3).

As Bernard continued to observe and experiment, it became evident that he was a physiologist of towering skill. He identified the two types of vasomotor nerves, characterized glycogen, and demonstrated how curare and carbon monoxide kill. He also developed the idea of homeostasis. "The theory of the constancy of the internal environment," wrote L. J. Henderson, "we owe almost wholly to Claude Bernard" (1961, viii). When Magendie retired, Bernard was appointed his successor.

Then, in 1860, when Bernard was forty-seven, disaster struck. Bernard developed diffuse, puzzling symptoms of some sort of debilitating disease. The symptoms became so bothersome that in 1862 he returned to his home in St. Julien to rest. Bernard's misfortune proved, however, to be a blessing for the rest of us, for the enforced rest gave him an opportunity to start a project he had thought about for a long time—a series of books on experimentation.

During the next two years he worked on the first volume, *An Introduction to the Study of Experimental Medicine*, which would, sadly, be the only one he would write. But that volume was a masterpiece.

"Nothing so complete, nothing so profound and so luminous," said his young friend, Louis Pasteur, "has ever been written on the true principles of the difficult art of experimentation. This book will exert an immense influence on medical science, its teaching, its progress, its language even. I seek in vain for a weak point in M. Bernard. It is not to be found" (Bender, 3).

Pasteur was right. The book would have enormous influence. For it was, in effect, a warning to physicians that unless they started thinking like chemists and physiologists, they were never going to get their patients well. Bernard had made an oblique reference to this point in the opening lecture of a series he gave at the College de France: "Scientific medicine, which it ought to be my duty to teach here, does not exist" (Bender, 4). But in 1865, when he published his book, he was able to say, "It is therefore clear to all unprejudiced minds that medicine is turning toward its permanent scientific path. [It is assuming] a more and more analytic form, and thus gradually [embracing] the method of investigation common to the experimental sciences" (Bernard 1961, xxi).

After recuperating for two years in St. Julien, Bernard returned to Paris. But he could no longer work as before. Three years later he returned to St. Julien, and in 1878, died. The government decreed that he have a state funeral, an honor never before accorded a scientist. Colleagues the world over, in one way or another, paid tribute to the man who had taught them so much about physiology and medicine. L. J. Henderson, with his characteristic economy of speech, summed up Claude Bernard's career in nine words: "His life was spent in putting questions to Nature."

The *Cahier Rouge*, the red notebook that Bernard kept for almost ten years, resembles a diary and contains, among other things, observations, ideas, and questions. Lots of questions: "In respiration is there a sort of digestion of air?" "Does blood losing water in a vacuum become red?" Sometimes there are volleys of questions, like, "Are all fishes capable of engendering a great quantity of ammonia as easily? Do fresh-water fishes have as numerous subcutaneous canals as marine fish? Is ammonia the cause of the viscous material which coats the body of fishes and prevents endosmosis by parts of the body other than the gills?"

Often, Bernard started with a fact, then jotted down questions the fact raised. For instance, "Nocturnal capillary hemorrhages of the buccal mucosa are arrested by crushed garlic. Could more serious hemorrhages be arrested? Does garlic exert a direct influence on the blood?"

Henri Bergson wrote that Bernard showed us how fact and idea "collaborate" in research. Research, Bergson said, is a dialogue between mind and nature. "Nature rouses our curiosity; we ask it questions; its answers give an unexpected turn to the conversation, starting new questions to which nature replies by suggesting new ideas" (1971, 239). The entries in the *Cahier Rouge* are splendid examples of this process.

But what, apart from grammatical form, makes a question different from a statement? What makes questions unique and indispensable? Is there, for instance, an advantage in asking, "Do the cells of the liver make glycogen?" rather than saying, "I'll bet the cells of the liver make glycogen." Yes, there is an advantage, and it lies, at least in part, in the different responses statements and questions evoke.

A statement may or may not stir us to action or even to active thinking, but being asked a question is like being near a telephone that's ringing: we feel compelled to answer both of them. And if we write a question down, rather than keep it in our head, we reap an extra benefit. For once a question's down on paper, we have a chance to see if it's in its clearest, simplest form. We can edit and revise it, just as we polish other kinds of writing. We may, in fact, need to revise it repeatedly, over several days. The sharper the question, the better the chance of finding an answer. The mind prefers crisp targets.

George Edward Moore stressed the importance of getting questions right when he wrote his small, durable textbook, *Principia Ethica* (1903). The opening sentence runs: "It appears to me that in Ethics, as in all other philosophical studies, the difficulties and disagreements of which history is full, are mainly due to a very simple cause: namely to the attempt to answer questions, without first discovering precisely *what* question it is which you desire to answer." Christopher Lasch, writing in *Harper's* on democracy, suggested a novel way to get questions right. He wrote,

> We do not know what we need to know until we ask the right questions, and we can identify the right questions only by subjecting our own ideas about the world to the test of public controversy. Information, usually seen as the precondition of debate, is better understood as its by-product. When we get into arguments that focus and really engage our attention, we become avid seekers of relevant information. Otherwise, we take in information passively—if we take it in at all. (1990, 17)

Certainly, Lasch's view holds for forums in clinical departments. Ideas set forth in public lead to debate and controversy, and eventually to questions. Then, the search for answers almost always sparks additional controversy. And this, in turn, sharpens the questions.

But what happens when we at last ask the right question, then start using the library or the laboratory to search for an answer? Popper has told us. Such a search, he says, inevitably raises additional questions that we can't answer. As a consequence, "our ignorance grows with our knowledge . . . and we shall therefore always have more questions than answers" (Magee, 31). What better way to insure continuing thought?

How, though, does the habit of asking questions in research laboratories spill over into other areas of a clinical department? Let me answer with a story. The late Hymie Nossel, a soft-spoken, scholarly member of the P and S faculty and an international authority on blood coagulation, seldom said much. Even so, interns and residents viewed Hymie as one of the best attending physicians on the staff. "Hymie," I said to him one day, "the house officers say you're one of the best attendings anywhere. But they also say you're as quiet on rounds as you are the rest of the time. What's your secret?"

Hymie thought for a moment, then said, "If the house officers want to know something, I ask myself, 'Do I know the answer?' If I do, I tell them. If I don't, I ask myself, 'Can I think of a way to get the answer?' If I can think of a way, I tell them. If I can't, there's no reason to say anything at all."

But when Hymie did speak, or ask himself questions, or share his questions with those around him, the interns and residents listened. They, like most young people, responded to logic.

# V

## Faculty, Students, Interns, and Residents

### *33*
### The Chair and the Faculty

Recruiting a faculty member is one of the hardest parts of a chair's job. No project is more important, and none is more likely to fail. The odds of success are better if the chair has decided to go for not-so-smart people (see section 4), rather than for people who are tops in their fields. Either way, the brightest feature of recruiting, especially for a new department, is that every person recruited increases the attractiveness of the department and makes the next recruitment easier.

Even when the job gets easier, recruiting is not a pastime one enjoys. Anyone doubting this should read Robert Petersdorf's account of it that he included in his presidential address to the Association of American Physicians (1977). Dr. Petersdorf took his listeners through the amenities of a candidate's visit—the plush hotel room, the flowers on the table, the wine, the dinners, the attention paid the candidate's spouse, and the demands for space, salary, and initial outlay of money (dowry) that candidates these days view as inalienable rights. "And, after the poor [chair] agreed to all," Bob said, "the candidate didn't accept."

The demand for a dowry is one of the biggest stumbling blocks to bringing in new people. In times past, a new faculty member, while waiting to get a grant, was given bench space and supplies by people already in the department. But now, a person being recruited demands up-front dollars with which to buy these things. In some instances, the department comes up with the dowry; in others, the dean helps out. Either way, the chair may have to pay a fearsome price, either in hard cash from his or her treasury or in IOUs to the dean.

A recruiting device that worked well for us at Stony Brook, and has worked well for other departments, is the intradepartmental search committee, a group of three or four people who operate like the schoolwide committees that look for deans and university presidents. We asked our committees to identify the best people and to eventually come up with two or three candidates for us to invite for visits. Once we had met the two or three and agreed on the one we wanted, the mating ritual described by Petersdorf began. Our batting average was fairly high, but then it should have been, because the State of New York had underwritten our school with extraordinary generosity.

Our recruiting, like recruiting everywhere, became more complex as the years went by, owing to new federal regulations, affirmative action guidelines, and, in some instances, state regulations that had to be followed when carrying out a search. At our school, the rules that cover searches for professional and nonprofessional personnel now fill a loose-leaf notebook more than an inch thick.

Occasionally a search has been much simpler. Burton (Bud) Pollack, a member of the staff at the Stony Brook dental school, was in his office one afternoon when Howard Oaks, vice president for health sciences, walked in and dropped into a chair. "Bud," Howie said, "I want you to be the new dean of the school of dental medicine." Bud made polite protests, then asked, "Why me?" "Because," Howie said, "I've talked to every member of the faculty, and you are the least disliked."

Once a search is completed and a faculty member recruited, what are the obligations of the chair? I doubt that any two chairs would give the same answer to this question, but all, I suspect, would say that one duty is to provide support. This means offering understanding and encouragement. It means letting new members know that the chair and the department will help them get where they hope to go. It means seeing that members get nominated for professional societies and for awards like Fulbrights and Guggenheims. And when the young faculty members receive an offer from another school, it means urging them to go take a look, while letting them know they are treasured at home.

Just as chairs have a range of opinions about their obligations to faculty members, so they have a range of ideas about the way members should be evaluated. Some chairs advocate once-a-year formal sessions, in which the chair reviews the member's performance, points out strengths and weaknesses, and discusses plans for the future. Other chairs have an informal meeting with each faculty member each year, a meeting in which the chair and member exchange ideas and opinions about the department and the member's role in it. And still others skip structured sessions of any sort. I served under Robert Loeb, Stanley Bradley, Charlie Ragan, and Dickinson Richards, and none ever held sessions like the ones just mentioned. Further, none of us on their staffs felt deprived.

The reason we didn't feel short-changed lies, I'm sure, in the fact that each of these leaders made himself continually available. Each maintained an open-door policy that invited ongoing talk. When, for instance, Charlie Ragan was chair at P and S, he would arrive early each morning, open the doors to his office, then keep them open for the next hour, as he sat at his desk and did paperwork. A knock was all that was needed to get an audience. In addition, Charlie, like the other three chairs, made it a habit to walk around the department almost every day and to stop for a brief chat with everyone he met. These men saw to it that their departments more closely resembled families than corporations, and with families, frequent informal chats are a better way to keep up to date than are structured talks.

If, on the other hand, a chair favors formal reviews and evaluations, he or she should read W. Edwards Deming's Deadly Disease #3, as set forth by Mary Walton (1986):

> *Evaluation by performance, merit rating or annual review of performance:* The effects of these are devastating—teamwork is destroyed, rivalry is nurtured. Performance ratings build fear and leave people bitter, despondent and beaten. (36)

Some chairs believe that they should train faculty members to run a department. David Weeks, chief of our division of general medicine and a pillar of our faculty, felt strongly about this. After finishing his residency, David worked for an American oil company in Saudi Arabia, a company with a training program that rotated junior people through administrative positions, leaving the person in each spot for the weeks or months necessary to get a feel for the job.

David would, from time to time, suggest that we try this in our department. We didn't. Perhaps we should have, but there was the worry that assignments such as supervising the department's ambulatory care service would take too much time away from research and other scholarly activities, things the oil company didn't need to worry about. We did try something else—a junior planning committee, advisory to the chair and to the department's advisory committee, made up of young faculty members. Each division elected an instructor or assistant professor to represent them, which gave the committee ten members. The ten then chose one of their number to chair their sessions and to make up agendas.

The planning committee met every two weeks for about two hours. The young people worked with great vigor and enthusiasm, researching each issue carefully, then putting the information together in their own way. Among the issues they chose to tackle were how to set salaries, how to divide practice money among the divisions, and what fraction of our hospital beds should be reserved for the patients of community physicians. Once the group had formed an opinion, they relayed it as a nonbinding recommendation to me and to our advisory committee. On occasion, a chief would decide that the young people were encroaching on his or her territory, and at these times, the chief would rail against the idea of a bunch of junior people digging into departmental business. But these incidents were infrequent, and, as time went by, I found the planning group an unending source of fresh ideas.

Thus far, I have talked about a chair's relation to faculty members in his or her own department. Now, a few words about the relation of a chair to the dean and to other chairs. In the dark hours of the soul—when, according to F. Scott Fitzgerald, it's always three o'clock in the morning—chairs have a built-in source of comfort: they can remind themselves that they aren't the dean. The dean has the hardest job in the medical school. A chair looks out for the people in his or her department, while a dean must look out for all of the people in all the departments. The dean must also ride herd on thirty or so clinical and basic science chairs, all mild to severe egocentrics, and try to keep them on a steady course. To do this requires patience, equanimity, resilience, and—most of all—common sense. The dean is the rock of the faculty, so much so that the faculty often reflects the dean's personality. Certainly this was true at Stony Brook, where all of us, in one way or another, reflected the personality of Marvin Kuschner, the ideal dean personified. A wise chair, of course, stays on good terms with the dean. A chair should also stay on good terms with as many other chairs as he or she can manage.

Back to faculties. Recently, there has been much talk, in both the lay and professional presses, about the future of clinical faculties. Predictions are that managed care will cause future faculties to be completely different from those in the past. I'm not sure about the *completely* part, but even now, in the midst of this revolution in medicine, when predictions made one day may be negated the next, a few things seem clear. One is that members of clinical departments will spend more time taking care of patients and planning care delivery systems than they have in the past. They will also need to spend more time building bridges between themselves and other clinical services and be more sensitive to the cost of care than they have been before.

An obvious effect of these expanded clinical activities will be that faculty members will have less time for research. But will constriction of time—and, maybe, dwindling funds—cause clinical investigators to disappear, as some prophets have predicted? No, I don't think they will, nor do I think that research in clinical departments will be taken over by Ph.D.s. It is important to remember that Ph.D.s have been in topnotch clinical departments for years and have made outstanding contributions to medicine, just as their M.D. colleagues have. But Ph.D. and M.D. researchers are not interchangeable, as some writers seem to think. Each type has its own unique view of medicine, and each has its own approach. Then too, dwindling research funds are going to hit Ph.D.s just as hard as M.D.s.

Some writers have said that faculties in the future will lay more emphasis on teaching. If these writers are implying that the quality of teaching will rise, then they are, I think, off base, because good teaching has been a primary goal of clinical departments since they came into existence. If, on the other hand, the writers mean that faculty members will receive more recognition for being good teachers, then I am with them. I am also with those who believe the meaning of tenure should be changed, so that achievements in teaching and patient care, as well as research, can be recognized and rewarded (see section 35).

In time, the upheavals caused by managed care will taper off, and clinical faculties will reach a new equilibrium. When this comes to pass, scholarship—in the form of research, writing, teaching, and clinical care—will still be around, despite the dire predictions we hear most every day. I hold this optimistic view even though I cannot predict the details of what will happen. But neither can those who prophesy doom.

## *34*

## Helpers versus Second-Guessers

Young faculty members feel compelled to criticize and protest, and in doing this they keep departments on their toes. But each young member should, at some time or other, switch to being a senior member, someone who takes responsibility for helping fix the things he or she complains about.

The process of switching, of growing and maturing, takes place in different ways. For most, the process is slow and steady. In others, it's dramatic, like the conversion of Sydney Carton. And in a few, the change is minimal, if there's any change at all. These few continue to criticize and protest, to jump up and down and shake their fists, sometimes at the world in general, more often at their chair. They view themselves as martyrs, crusading for high standards. But in the eyes of friends and colleagues, such people are adolescents, doomed to second-guess forever.

Nonswitchers not only damage themselves but infect those around them. "New data," wrote Daniel Goleman in the *New York Times* in 1991, "depict moods as akin to social viruses, with some people having a natural ability to transmit them while others are more susceptible to contagion." Goleman then quotes Elaine Hatfield, a psychologist at the University of Hawaii. Dr. Hatfield reported, at the meeting of the American Psychological Society in June 1991, that "emotional contagion happens within milliseconds, so quickly you can't control it, and so subtly that you're not really aware it's going on."

One mechanism at work in the transmission of moods, Goleman continues, "is the tendency of people to imitate the expressions of faces they look at. For example, Swedish researchers reported in 1986 that when people viewed pictures of smiling or angry faces, their facial muscles changed slightly to mimic those faces. . . . While the changes were fleeting, and not visible to the eye, they were detected using electrodes that measured electrical activity in the muscles."

A clue that a young faculty member has made the switch is that he or she stops using superlatives when filing a complaint. This discovery came to me at a time when I fancied that my taste in literature was improving. I had noticed that I more and more enjoyed lean, uncluttered prose. Then I realized that my improved taste was, in reality, a reaction to the world of superlatives in which I lived. The young men and women who came to me to complain did so in the most extreme terms: "This is the worst . . . ." "Morale has hit bottom." "Everybody's going to quit." After making the transition, the young people spoke in less florid terms.

It is important to distinguish immature people from the young men and women who sit home nights, thinking about the department, absolutely sure they could run it better than the chair does. The thoughts of the latter spring from self-confidence and logic, the thoughts of the immature from resentment.

It is also important to distinguish immature people from department members who have made the switch but think differently from others. "Any organization," Peter Drucker says, "needs a nonconformist. . . . You don't want only yes-men and yes-women."

Nonconformists can also serve as the loyal opposition. In clinical departments, you don't need opposition like, say, the Labor party in the British Parliament, a group that often seems dedicated to knocking down whatever the Tories suggest. But opposition of some sort is essential in any organization. "No government," said Disraeli, "can be long secure without a formidable Opposition." Nonconformists play this role.

The fine line between being a useful or destructive critic, a traitorous or loyal faculty member, is difficult to walk, because it's often hard to think independently and at the same time be loyal to the department and the school.

Twenty-four hundred years ago, the Greeks faced a similar dilemma. Edith Hamilton said that "the Athenian was a law unto himself, but his dominant instinct to stand alone was counterbalanced by his sense of overwhelming obligation to serve the state. . . . The city was his defense in a hostile world, his security, his pride" (1942, 225). Then Ms. Hamilton tells us where our word *idiot* comes from. It comes from the name the Greeks gave people who stood alone, accepting the protection of their government but refusing to take part in the affairs of their city-state.

## 35
## The Credits and Debits of Tenure

Although the early history of tenure is clouded, we know that the idea of protecting scholars existed in the Middle Ages, four hundred years before Machiavelli wrote *The Prince*. "As early as 1158, the Emperor Frederick Barbarossa issued an edict promising scholars in his domains safe conduct in their journeys, protection from attack upon their domiciles, and compensation for unlawful injury . . . [from] country brigands and city mobs" (Metzger 1973, 94). And protection, as everyone knows, remains the bedrock feature of tenure today.

But other aspects of tenure have changed. The principal enemies, for instance, are no longer brigands and mobs, but chairs, deans, vice presidents, chancellors, trustees, and other administrators who—academics are certain—may cut their salaries, block their promotions, or even force their dismissal if the academics cross them.

A second change is that tenure is now linked to salary. This change can be dated to 1940, when the American Association of University Professors and the Association of American Colleges issued a joint statement that first underscored the need for continued academic freedom, then called for "a sufficient degree of economic security to make the profession attractive to men and women of ability." Thus, the joint statement added the idea of salary to the original idea of freedom.

In the fifty years that have gone by since the two associations drafted their statement, the concept of tenure has continued to grow. Today, a tenure package may include protected speech, a permanent appointment, a permanent faculty title, eligibility for sabbatical leave, and a salary that will continue until retirement, barring the financial collapse of the university or the school. Hence, tenure, in the eyes of most faculty members, confers priceless benefits. It also confers a priceless honor: a ringing vote of confidence.

Yet, questions about tenure, in both medical and nonmedical parts of universities, are continually raised, sometimes by administrators who dislike the independence of tenured people, sometimes by academics who view the system as pernicious, and sometimes by nonacademics who complain that tenured professors give teaching short shrift, thus imposing an economic burden on taxpayers. So let's begin by looking at some of the questions about tenure generally, not just tenure in medical schools.

### Is it true that tenured professors are completely independent, that they have no boss?

Henry Rosovsky, formerly dean of the Faculty of Arts and Sciences at Harvard, speaks to this point in his engaging book *The University: An Owner's Manual* (1990).

Another critical virtue of academic life—I am thinking of tenured professors at, say, America's top fifty to one hundred institutions—is the absence of a boss. A boss is someone who can tell you what to do, and requires you to do it—an impairment of freedom. As a dean—i.e., as an administrator—my boss was the president [of Harvard]. . . . But as a professor, I recognized no master save peer pressure, no threat except, perhaps, an unlikely charge of moral turpitude. (163–64)

I'm not sure people in medical schools view tenure quite this way. My guess is that tenured members of a medical faculty would say they had a boss—probably their chair—for even though it is the university, not the department, that grants tenure, the chair usually controls the space used by tenured people, as well as their salaries. Chairs in medical schools are able to do this because they tend to hold office longer and wield more power than chairs in other parts of universities. Also, I doubt that members of medical faculties think that winning tenure frees them from departmental duties.

### Why do some academics object to tenure?

David Helfand, a member of the Department of Physics at Columbia University, presented a typical argument against tenure.

> I turned down tenure, because I believe that the university tenure system should be abolished. Tenure is rooted in the premise that academic freedom and review of performance are somehow antithetical. It is, however, more often used to deprive young academics of freedom than to defend the senior faculty it is designed to protect. It can exclude productive, energetic scholars . . . maintain unproductive, unmotivated teachers . . . and discourage our best young minds from pursuing academic careers. (1986, 33)

Helfand added that the tenure system also attracts and protects "faculty members more concerned about preserving their job security than in defending their convictions."

### Can tenured professors stuff the roster of a department and thus prevent the infusion of new people?

Yes. And this can kill a department. In some schools, especially state schools, 90 percent of the people may be tenured, which means departments have little chance to bring in new recruits with fresh ideas.

### How about the fairness of the "tenure clock?"

In a typical school that has a tenure clock (also known as an up-or-out plan), the clock starts when a person joins the faculty. Then, unless the person receives credit for time spent at another school, the clock gives the person six years to acquire the credentials needed for tenure. During the sixth year, a committee reviews the credentials, decides whether to recommend tenure, and, if the answer is yes, forwards the recommendation to the chancellor. If the chancellor concurs, the person becomes tenured at the start of the seventh year. But if either the committee or the chancellor votes against tenure, the person is expected to leave the school by the end of the seventh year.

Though the plan is straightforward, it can, in a clinical department, be subverted in several ways. If, for instance, the work of a person on a research track proves to be less than satisfactory, the chair may shift the person from the research track to the clinical track, and request that the committee review the person for clinical tenure. Another tactic used for people whose research is progressing slowly is for the chair to ask the dean to change the person's appointment to a non-tenure-generating title, thereby stopping the tenure clock. Then, when the person has strengthened his or her credentials, the chair changes the title back again. A third twist is sometimes used with people who have been turned down for tenure. Instead of insisting that the person go elsewhere by the end of the seventh year, the chair, with the dean's concurrence, gives the person a nontenure generating title, then lets the person stay on indefinitely by using renewable temporary appointments.

These subterfuges are not necessarily fair or unfair, so long as they are available to everyone in the school. But a subterfuge becomes unfair when it is applied on a personal or departmental basis, rather than schoolwide. This should not happen if the rules are clearly stated, and if the dean, or someone the dean appoints, enforces the rules.

*How ironclad is the protection provided by tenure?*

The usual answer, as Rosovsky says, is that a tenured person is safe unless he or she commits some sort of grave offense, like being dishonest or being guilty of moral dereliction. But in the 1950s, Sen. Joseph McCarthy put tenure to a different and more stringent test. McCarthy vowed to expose closet "communists and pinkos," especially in universities. He was, he declared, certain that universities harbored lots of them.

Did tenure afford protection against McCarthy's deadly attacks? No. Both tenured and nontenured professors were fired for their political views. This happened because the decisions lay in the hands of ruling boards, and some boards wilted under the fierce glare of McCarthy's televised hearings. Hence, the traditional view that tenure provides ironclad protection is an illusion.

As mentioned, the questions just considered deal with tenure generally. Now, we shall turn to tenure for medical faculties, especially the faculties of clinical departments.

In 1982 Smythe, Jones, and Wilson, faculty members at Houston, Albany, and Maryland, respectively, wrote a paper entitled "Tenure in Medical Schools in the 1980s." The authors based their discussion on the belief that the rapid growth in the size, number, and programs of medical schools that occurred in the 1960s and 1970s had ended and that tenure, in the new era of slowed growth, would have to undergo changes. They mentioned changes that might occur in the appointment process, and they deemed those changes a "healthy evolutionary process." In their summary and conclusions, Smythe and his colleagues said: "Despite the somewhat circuitous processes implied, the rewards of having a faculty solidly in support of tenure policies are so great as to justify deep involvement of the faculty in alterations in appointment systems. . . . In the final analysis, tenure is a manageable process" (359).

Two years later, Robert Petersdorf expressed a different view. In a paper entitled "The Case against Tenure in Medical Schools" (1984), he built a compelling case for dropping tenure for medical faculties. Among his arguments were that universities were saddled with an aging, expensive cadre of tenured faculty members and that the cadre had tied up university funds; that these faculty members, in Dr. Petersdorf's experience, often slacked off or became "disengaged"; that political pressures, like those that had brought tenure into existence, were by then seldom seen and if they did occur could be handled by grievance committees; that a faculty member granted tenure for excellence at, say, 35 or 40, might not remain excellent; and that clinical departments were heavily dependent on good practitioners, yet tenure committees seldom recognized this fact. Dr. Petersdorf suggested substituting renewable contracts for tenure. He also pointed out that dropping tenure would enable clinical departments to simplify their system of academic titles and use just assistant, associate, and full professor.

My view of tenure in clinical departments lies between that of Smythe, Jones, and Wilson and that of Petersdorf. For me, the most worrisome feature of tenure in clinical departments is that it may not be equally available to all department members. As Dr. Petersdorf said, people doing research are much more likely to win tenure than those who do clinical work, even though a modern department is as dependent on clinicians as it is on investigators. Schools that have tackled the problem by creating special tenure tracks for clinical people have found that system hard to implement. Take, for instance, the matter of publications. Academic clinicians should publish, just as researchers do, because contributing to our store of knowledge is, after all, the mark of the academician. But how many papers in what journals should a tenure committee demand?

Another hitch in a clinical track has been that clinicians are usually judged heavily on their ability as teachers, as if they had a corner on teaching. This emphasis conflicts with the longstanding belief that everyone in a clinical department, researcher as well as clinician, should work to become a skilled teacher. It goes without saying that the better the teacher, the better the case for tenure; but this should hold for everyone, researchers and clinicians alike. In short, using teaching as a discriminator is a bad idea.

A third problem with the clinical track is that it adds still another definition of tenure. Tenure for a research person rests on research first, then patient care and teaching; tenure for a clinical person rests first on patient care, followed by research and teaching; and tenure for a basic scientist rests on research and then on teaching. The principal criterion in each sequence is, incidentally, the area where the person excels, the skill that the tenure committee will scrutinize most closely. The practical importance of the sequences is that members of tenure committees have to cope with three different sets of standards, all ephemeral and imprecise.

An attractive feature of the contracts that Petersdorf advocated was the possibility that they would free tenure committees from having to deal with all the baggage that over the last 800 years has become attached to the word *tenure*. Committee members could stop picturing a tenured person as a single type, a man or woman who does research, has a long bibliography, belongs to learned societies, and has a reputation that is at least nationwide. Committees might even begin by assessing a candidate's worth to the school and department, rather than the merit of his or her personal achievements. The committee might ask questions like: Is the candidate important to the long-term mission and goals of the school and department? Has the candidate switched from being a junior to a senior department member, to being a person willing to take responsibility for the way the school and department run (see section 34)? Afterward, the committee could tackle the daunting task of judging research and clinical skill.

There are, of course, ways of rewarding clinicians other than tenure. Some schools have allowed clinicians to make higher salaries or to have more indirect costs. These remedies are fine for clinical chairs who aren't bothered by being able to bestow nonmonetary honors on some of their people and not on others, but these remedies won't work for chairs who deem this unfair.

I would vote for keeping tenure in clinical departments, *provided the inequities just mentioned can be abolished.* If this can be done, then tenure could be defended on the basis of free speech alone, without invoking frills like salaries and sabbaticals.

The goal of a clinical faculty should be to make tenure work. To this end, a clinical faculty might approach tenure in the way Mark Van Doren believed faculties should approach liberal education. Liberal education would work, Van Doren said, only if we give it our best thought and argument, "argument, that is to say, about the greatest things, the difficult, the all but insoluble things that haunt us every morning as we wake" (1959, iii). And if, when approached in this way, the inequities can be abolished, tenure should be continued. But if the inequities cannot be abolished, tenure—at least in clinical departments—should be dropped.

## *36*
## Why Faculty Titles Need to Be Changed

Just as there are inequities in the criteria for tenure, so there are inconsistencies in our academic titles. Not only inconsistencies, but, in the eyes of many faculty members, unfairness, for some titles are considered prestigious while others are thought to be demeaning. I shall talk first about the inconsistencies, and though it may seem quaint and antiquated, I shall begin by reviewing the titles the U.S. Navy gave reserve officers in World War II. Back then, a college graduate entering officer training went to one of two types of midshipman schools: deck (D) or engineering (E). The brand new officers who emerged three months later were titled, respectively, "Ensign (D)" and "Ensign (E)." Each title combined the rank, Ensign, with a descriptor, D or E. These were the official titles, the ones on the rolls of the Bureau of Personnel. But on informal rosters the descriptors were omitted. You would not, however, see on any one document some titles with descriptors and others without. The navy liked consistency.

In a clinical department, members teach, help with administration, take care of patients, and do research. But since everyone teaches and helps with administration, the descriptors that separate people, the counterparts of *deck* and *engineering*, are *clinical* and *research*. One might, therefore, expect to see two types of titles: professor of clinical and professor of research. And though every school, I guess, has the equivalent of the title professor of clinical, few have professors of research. Instead, they have just plain professors. Medical schools, unlike the navy, aren't big on consistency.

Consistency wasn't a problem in the days when every salaried member of a clinical department did research. Each person had one of the unmodified titles: assistant professor, associate professor, or professor. Titles with *clinical* in them were given to unsalaried faculty members, physicians who practiced in the community and who helped teach students, interns, and residents. Thus, the word *clinical* separated full-time, salaried faculty members from part-time volunteers.

But when departments of family medicine and divisions of general medicine came into existence, faculties acquired full-time, salaried clinicians, and these people needed titles. If they, like the researchers, were given unmodified titles, they would have to be held to the same standards for promotion and tenure as the researchers, which would mean lots of papers, memberships, and all the rest. And being chiefly involved in patient care, the clinicians would not be able to produce many of these things. So, to get around the problem, schools gave full-time, salaried clinical people titles with *clinical* in them.

This solved one problem but created another. The new problem was that full-time clinicians disliked the idea of having the same titles as part-time volunteers. And even when schools put *clinical* in one place in titles for full-time people (professor of clinical) and in another place for part-time people (clinical professor of), the full-time people stayed upset. Any title with *clinical* in it sparked resentment in full-time staff members. As the years have gone by, this unhappiness with titles has grumbled along.

The simplest remedy, it seems to me, is to do for full-time people what the navy did for its officers and what some deans have done, namely, give each new faculty member an official title with either *clinical* or *research* in it. This would be the title that would appear in university records and on the person's curriculum vitae. But then the dean should hide the official titles and tell members of the faculty—clinical and research people alike—that when they write letters, submit abstracts, publish papers, or do other such things, they should all use unmodified titles: assistant, associate, or professor.

This scheme isn't perfect. It will, most likely, irk the researchers who believe the unmodified title should belong only to them. But researchers, as well as everyone else, should understand that a professor is a professor is a professor, whether he or she takes care of patients, does research, or teaches integral calculus.

It comes down to this: A chair who doesn't worry about clinical people being unhappy can vote for keeping the clinical and unmodified titles, the two series now in general use; tradition will be on his or her side. But a chair who considers clinicians and researchers equally important and worries about unfairness will lobby for another system, a system with titles clinicians will be proud of, just as researchers are proud of theirs.

The navy's scheme should accomplish this. Friends who've tried similar schemes say they work.

## *37*

## Flatterers and Counselors

"I will not leave unnoticed," Machiavelli wrote, "an important subject, and an evil against which princes have much difficulty in defending themselves . . . and this relates to flatterers, who abound in all courts. Men are generally so well pleased with themselves . . . and delude themselves to such a degree . . . that it is with difficulty they escape from the pest of flatterers; and in their efforts to avoid them, they expose themselves to the risk of being scorned" (105).

The flattery Machiavelli talked about was most likely the type that has been with us always. We tell a young poet she writes like Emily Dickinson, or say to a freshman senator that he speaks like Winston Churchill. This sort of flattery has the virtue of being obvious. It can be easily recognized. But there is another, more pernicious type of flattery that is harder to deal with. G. K. Chesterton wrote about it near the turn of the present century.

There has crept into our literature and journalism a new way of flattering the wealthy and the great. In more straightforward times flattery was itself more straightforward; falsehood itself was more true. . . . When courtiers sang the praises of a King they attributed to him things that were entirely improbable, as that he resembled the sun at noonday, that they had to shade their eyes when he entered the room. The safety of this method was its artificiality; between the King and his public image there was really no relation. . . . [People today] have invented a much subtler and more poisonous kind of eulogy. The modern method is to take the prince or rich man, to give a credible picture of his type of personality, as he is business-like, or a sportsman, or fond of art, or convivial, or reserved; and then enormously exaggerate the value and importance of these natural qualities. Those who praise Mr. Carnegie do not say he is as wise as Solomon. . . . I wish they did. . . . What they do is to take the rich man's superficial life and manner, clothes, hobbies, love of cats, dislike of doctors, or what not; and then with the assistance of this realism make the man out to be a prophet and a saviour of his kind. (133–34)

This second kind of flattery, like the first, must be recognized and dealt with.

Machiavelli said that the best way to guard against adulation is to obviate the need for it by letting people know they will not offend you by speaking the truth. Chairs who take this advice will ask members of their departments for opinions but will, at the same time, be wary of what the members say. Faculty members cannot help flattering the chair, either consciously or subconsciously, because they like the chair, fear the chair, or need something the chair alone can give.

But there is another way to get advice and counsel, a way secure from flatterers, and that is to study what great men and women have said and written in the past. Machiavelli did this, especially after the Medicis returned to power and banned him to a villa outside Florence. Here, he had time for study and reflection, and in a letter to his friend, Vettori, Machiavelli described the way he spent his days.

When he got up each morning, Machiavelli took a walk in the woods and talked to the woodcutters. Then he found a spot on a hill, sat down, and read Dante or Petrarch or Ovid. After a small lunch, he went to the inn to talk to friends—the butcher, the bricklayer, and the miller. And he often spent the rest of the afternoon playing cards with "boors."

> But when evening comes, I return to the house and go into my study. Before I enter I take off my rough mud-stained country dress. I put on my royal and curial robes and thus fittingly attired I enter into the assembly of men of old times. Welcomed by them I feed upon that food which is my true nourishment, and which has made me what I am. I dare to talk with them and ask them the reasons for their actions. Of their kindness they answer me. . . . From these notes I have composed a little work, *The Prince*. (Gauss 1980, 11)

Every chair, with a bit of thought, will be able to jot down the names of a dozen or so books that have provided the sort of nourishment Machiavelli mentioned. Some of the books will be practical, how-to books. Others will be theoretical, what-is-the-case books. But regardless of the type, each will, in all probability, be a book that will have to be read in small chunks, with frequent time-outs to absorb the message in the paragraph just finished.

The books will be like *A Discourse on Method*, René Descartes; *An Essay Concerning Human Understanding*, John Locke; *An Introduction to the Study of Experimental Medicine*, Claude Bernard; *Enquiry Concerning the Understanding*, David Hume; *Essays*, Michel Eyquem de Montaigne; *How to Read a Book*, Mortimer Adler and Charles Van Doren; *Karl Popper*, Bryan Magee; *Liberal Education*, Mark Van Doren; *Lives of a Cell*, and anything else Lewis Thomas has written; *Macbeth*, and anything else Shakespeare wrote; *Meno*, Plato; *Objective Knowledge: An Evolutionary Approach*, Karl Popper; *Physics and Philosophy*, Werner Heissenberg; *Science and Method*, Henri Poincaré; *The Cahier Rouge of Claude Bernard*, Hebbel Hoff, Lucienne Guillemin, and Roger Guillemin; *The Logic of Scientific Discovery*, Karl Popper; *The New Organum*, Francis Bacon; *Two Treatises on Government*, John Locke; and *What Is Life?* Irwin Schroedinger.

Few of these books are directly connected to medicine, yet connections are there. Open, for example, the small paperback, *What Is Life?* and turn to the page where Erwin Schroedinger, the physicist who won a Nobel Prize for his work on wave mechanics, talks about Fick's Law of Diffusion. Few educators, professional or otherwise, have explained a first-order partial differential equation with such overwhelming clarity. Schroedinger gives all of us a lesson in how to teach.

A number of the books provide counsel of a different sort: they tell us how people behave. To learn about everyday human behavior, a person might read Shakespeare. Then, maybe, Freud. But Shakespeare first. For great poetry and literature, Cleanth Brooks says, "let us observe and overhear men and women as they choose, make decisions, or express their inmost hopes and fears. That in itself is a service of the utmost importance, for we can learn from the experience of others."

This service, Brooks continues, "rendered by the great literature throughout history . . . provides dramatic accounts of men and women in conflict with nature and with other human beings, and often with themselves. This last conflict . . . the tug between two loyalties, two evils, or what appear to be two equally precious goods—is probably the most instructive of all. Sophocles' *Antigone* and his *Oedipus*, Shakespeare's *Othello*, *Macbeth* and *Mark Antony*, are only a few of an illustrious company." The conflicts Brooks mentions, and the sense of helplessness that comes when a person can't resolve them, lie at the heart of the practice of psychiatry.

In addition to books, there is another source of counsel, also immune from flattery, that all of us use instinctively. It is reflection on the thoughts and actions of wise men and women we ourselves have known. We are forever listening to voices from the past, voices of parents, teachers, and wise friends. And clinical chairs listen especially to voices of the great leaders they have known, for nothing is more comforting when a hard problem arises than to be able to pause and ask one's self, "What would he or she have done?"

Machiavelli acknowledged his debt to counselors when, at the beginning of *The Prince*, he dedicated the book to Lorenzo the Magnificent: "I have found nothing that I hold more dear or esteem more highly than the knowledge of the actions of great men, which I have acquired by long experience of modern affairs, and a continued study of ancient history."

Most of us, I'll bet, feel the same way.

## 38
## Students, Interns, and Residents

The obligations of a chair to students, interns, and residents fall into three broad categories: teaching, counseling, and making sure the medical school curriculum provides the best training possible. A chair may, of course, help young colleagues in other ways, but teaching, counseling, and checking the curriculum are by far the most important ones.

### Teaching

Nobody has discussed the student-teacher contract with more charm and clarity than Mark Van Doren in his small book *Liberal Education* (1959). And though Van Doren focused on the liberal arts, his insights apply with equal force to teaching and learning medicine (Fritts, 1977). Van Doren's thoughts about what to teach were simple and direct.

> The notion persists that [the student] is the chief concern of education. In one sense he certainly is: we want all the individuals we can get, and we want the best ones possible. But it remains a real question how we get them; I suspect it is not by trimming education to what is supposed to be their individual needs. I continue to believe that the way to produce individual intellects is to teach all students the same things, and of course the best things. They will make their own responses, and discover their own ideas; but these will be best when the material for study has been the kind of material that is good for everybody. (vi)

What are the best things a clinical department can offer? One possibility is a collection of facts. Facts are necessary for the practice of medicine and are critically important for students taking National Boards. Yet, Van Doren doubted the wisdom of stressing factual material and, in discussing the matter, offered the following advice:

> As little attention as possible will be wasted on details of knowledge which the student is certain to forget. Such of them as point a principle need to be mastered, but then if a right relation is maintained between detail and principle, the detail will not be forgotten. It will become an item in the mind around which other details organize themselves as long as life lasts. (8)

The principles a clinical department might teach include the steps suggested by A. M. Harvey and J. Bordley (1970) for analyzing clinical data, P. A. Tumulty's method (1973, 189–99) for making diagnoses, and W. P. Harvey's five-finger technique (1964) for evaluating patients with heart disease. Principles like these retain their value; facts have a habit of becoming obsolete.

I have, incidentally, wondered whether teaching principles might explain a comment Dr. Yale Kneeland made when chairing a combined clinic at P and S thirty years ago. "I never cease to marvel," he said, "how year after year we manage to teach medical students more than we ourselves know." Teaching principles can do this. Teaching facts cannot.

Van Doren believed the goals of education should be to discipline the mind, to equip it to solve problems, to strip it of prejudice, to leave it free to do its work.

> When we go to a wise man for advice it is not to learn what he knows about everything; it is to benefit by what he knows about the single thing that troubles us. If he seems to bring vast considerations to bear upon it, well and good; we should scarcely be comfortable otherwise; but what we want in the end is his opinion as to here, to now, to this. The surest proof that any mind is free is its faith in itself when faced with hard questions. It may not be sure that it can answer them but it does not doubt its capacities to make the attempt. (iii)

These lines come close to describing the way expert clinicians think and work. By mastering principles, they acquire such self-assurance that regardless of the complexity of the problems they encounter, they know how to begin.

Then Van Doren talks about the student's responsibility in the educational process.

> Much of the burden in education is safely left where it belongs, on the back of the students. Faculties are asked what they can do for boys and girls who come to them to "get" an education, and they have fallen into the habit of enumerating the things they will "give," as if a list were all. When education goes wrong, the subject of it is partly to blame. This is not said often enough or firmly enough for the young to heed it. . . . Teaching helps, and it should be as good as possible. But there is also the person to be taught, and he should have the desire no less than the ability. (6–7)

Twenty-four centuries earlier, Aeschylus, in *Agamemnon*, had written about the learner's role in learning and about the price the learner pays: "God, whose law it is that he who learns must suffer. And even in our sleep pain that cannot forget, falls drop by drop upon the heart, and in our own despite, against our will, comes wisdom to us by the awful grace of God." Thus, Aeschylus, like Van Doren, stressed the heavy responsibility the student carries in the student-teacher partnership.

Whenever someone mentions the bond between students and teachers, I think back to a day in the 1950s when Bill Briscoe, a member of the Cardio-Pulmonary Laboratory at Bellevue Hospital, told us that he planned to visit northern England. On hearing this, André Cournand, the director of the laboratory, asked Bill to see if he could locate the former headmaster of the school Cournand had attended in his early teens. The man had retired to northern England and become a recluse, so his acquaintances in the States had lost track of him. André wasn't sure the teacher would remember him and suggested that Bill mention that Cournand had played football.

When Bill Briscoe reached northern England, he found the old man, almost deaf and almost blind. Bill asked if he remembered André Cournand, one of his boys from long ago. "Sure, I remember André," the old headmaster said. "Played football. Fiercest football player I ever saw. If André tackled a man and the man got up, André would knock him down again."

The old man was silent for a moment, then said, "From time to time, I've wondered what became of André." Bill told him that the previous year Cournand had been awarded the Nobel Prize in medicine. The old man let this sink in and then said, "No, . . . no, that would have had to be a different André Cournand."

## Counseling

The word *counseling* has a bad connotation these days, because we usually hear it in connection with someone who's misbehaved and needs straightening out. But a more important type of counseling takes place, for instance, when a chair helps students, interns, and residents decide about the places they want to go. For students, this entails talking to them, discussing the various types of internships, then helping them get the internships they would like to have. And for interns and residents, it means helping them get into the training programs they would like to join, or helping them get appointed to the staffs of hospitals where they would like to practice medicine.

There is another type of counseling that can be overt or subliminal. It entails letting young people know what it means to be a physician. A fine way to start is to suggest that they read what Dr. D. W. Richards had to say about the matter in his 1962 presidential address at the Association of American Physicians. The address, among other things, highlights the parts of medical practice that our growing technology cannot replace.

Once a physician takes upon himself the responsibility for a patient's care, instantly he becomes a different man. In identifying himself thus with medicine as a profession, he accepts a social discipline. He must define the problem anew, for himself and for everyone, for each particular situation in each particular case: Precisely what is my responsibility here? Who takes care of what I do not take care of? Does this other fellow know about it? . . . If ever there were an all-or-none law, it is in patient care.

The reason for this is as old as time, that human suffering, in its vast and multitudinous complexity, has always this in common, that it pervades the whole sick man, and this whole must be cared for. Suffering, moreover, is different from misfortune: it comes not in battalions but by one and one. Each man's is his own. If you would know about human suffering, study your patient, as he lies there, as he looks at you, his eyes, his voice, how he moves, what he says, how he says it. Then from here you build up the whole structure of your care, a broad structure, as broad as the measure of his distress. Surely this is no denial of medical science, but its fulfillment. There is no need to argue this in this audience; it has been exemplified by the great clinicians of the Association over all these five and seventy years.

Hippocrates said it more clearly, and more briefly, than anyone. You will remember his sober words: "It is necessary," said he, "for the physician to provide not only the needed treatment, but to provide for the sick man himself, and for those beside him, and to provide for his outside affairs." This is a large order, but this is what Hippocrates has said, and one must agree that he is right. (9)*

Richards is a fine mentor when a chair must counsel students, interns, or residents on what it means to be a physician. But then Richards is a fine mentor for a chair at any time.

## Monitoring the Medical School Curriculum

Ludwig Eichna is in the best position of anyone I know to comment on the curriculum we use for training medical students. Dr.

---

*Excerpts reprinted by permission of *Proceedings of the Association of American Physicians* (formerly *Transactions of the Association of American Physicians*) and Blackwell Science, Inc.

Eichna, after a distinguished career as chair of medicine at Down-state Medical Center in New York, enrolled as a student and went through medical school again. He did this because "for a number of years before retirement" he had been "increasingly dissatisfied with the course and results of medical school education." He could not, however, pinpoint the source of his dissatisfaction. The only way to do this, he decided, would be to go through the course of training himself. So after retiring in July 1974, he became a full-time student at Downstate in September 1975. He later described his unusual choice in an article in the *New England Journal of Medicine*.*

> I made the decision to take everything that regular medical students went through, including lectures, conferences, seminars, reports, lab-oratories, patient workups and presentations, operating room and de-livery room duties, nights and weekends on call, and all examinations, written and oral, including National Boards Part I and Part II. . . . All contact with faculty and administration, aside from scheduled teach-ing activities, was completely severed. The result was acceptance by students as one of them, not a dean's-office "plant," not a "company man." An easy relationship of equality resulted. Students expressed their thoughts freely. It was essential to know how students felt, for my own reactions could be different, influenced by a past experience that could not be erased. (1980, 727)

Ike finished with the class of 1979. He then turned to the diaries and journals he had kept during his days as a student, and wrote the account of his experiences. The paper, packed with insights, tells us about both the bad features of medical training and the parts that are good. From his experience, Dr. Eichna developed eight basic principles for medical education. Although he called them obvious, he found that each principle was "routinely violated." Here are his principles.

*Excerpts reprinted by permission of *The New England Journal of Medicine* and the Massachusetts Medical Society.

Principle 1. The focus and first priority of medical-school education is the patient.

Principle 2. The profession of medicine is a science, humanely conducted.

Principle 3. Learning is a thinking, problem-solving process that requires time.

Principle 4. Medical education is a continuum, binding college education, medical-school education, and postgraduate house-officership training into a unified whole.

Principle 5. Learning medicine requires a proper balance of apprenticeship (practical) training and formal teaching in lectures and seminars.

Principle 6. Education requires evaluation procedures that correctly assess progress and competence.

Principle 7. Medical school education requires adherence to a standard of excellence.

Principle 8. The profession of medicine demands at all levels, specifically including that of medical students, the highest ethical conduct.

Ike wrote long paragraphs about each of the principles, paragraphs that are a must-read for anyone in medical education. He details the reasons the principles sometimes get ignored and tells us how to avoid such lapses.

Near the end of his paper, Ike wrote the following lines:

We are not industrialists. We do not conduct a business. We sell no product to consumers. We are doctors. We take care of, and we care for, patients. We must be mindful of cost, yes, but the patient comes first.

Ike was prescient. His blunt statements, written sixteen years ago, crytallize the dilemma that physicians face today.

## 39

## Why Chairs Must Be Periodically Replaced and Faculties Periodically Renewed

"It passes my persimmon," Osler said, "to tell how some good men—even lovable and righteous men in other respects—have the hardihood to stay in the same position for twenty-five years" (1974, 377). I know what Osler meant, because I, like the people Osler mentioned, stayed in office too long. My fifteen years were, as our British colleagues might put it, too many by half.

There's no magic number of years a clinical chair should serve, but my hunch is that the average person should hold the job for seven to ten years. This is enough time for a chair to get done what he or she hopes to get done, if the chair aspires to be more than a caretaker. And for those who dislike the seven-to-ten-year suggestion, a good rule to follow is the one we've heard forever, "quit while you're ahead." For a clinical chair, this means quitting while the department is flourishing.

But that's when chairs are least likely to quit. The department is successful, chairs will tell themselves, so why not sit back and enjoy what their efforts have wrought? But departments don't stay successful—they eventually slide downhill. And a chair who waits to retire until after the slide begins is in for an unhappy time.

A few years ago, a chair of medicine whom I know stepped down while his department was thriving. Six months later, when he needed his cholesterol checked, he visited the emergency room in his university's hospital, a place he had frequented for all the years he had been a chair. The reception had been overwhelming, he told friends later. The staff members had said things like, "We wish you were back," "We talk about you all the time," and "We remember how you had the interns and residents wear ties." The ex-chair was surprised, and he wondered if the reception would have been so warm if he had resigned earlier, when the department had been "in the dumps." He decided it wouldn't have been, and he concluded, "People seem to remember you for the way you were at the finish."

Any discussion of replacing chairs brings into focus the nature of clinical departments and the process they use to change their leaders. Are departments autocracies, democracies, or something else? Those with absolute chairs can be autocracies, for in those departments, the chair's word is law. But departments with liberal chairs cannot be full democracies—not, at least, in the usual sense of the word. They can, it is true, confer civil rights—guarantees of free speech and free expression—but they cannot confer political rights, that is, permission to form an alternative government with a leader who can replace the chair. Instead, a search committee chooses the new chair for them.

So, department members who persuade a dean to fire a chair are gambling. They have to hope that whoever the search committee comes up with will be better than the chair who's being fired.

From time to time, someone suggests that members of a department should choose new chairs, rather than letting a search committee do it. I'm not sure this would be a good idea. Experts on management tell us that when an organization needs a new head, the people making the selection should avoid a carbon copy of the old leader. Search committees would, I think, be more apt to follow this advice than members of a department would.

And just as chairs need to be replaced from time to time, so members of departments need changing too. People who work together, we are told, begin to think alike after about four years. Hence, a department that doesn't infuse itself with new people risks stagnation.

Henry Ford held strong views about workers who stay in jobs too long. "It isn't the incompetent who destroy an organization," he said. "The incompetent never get into a position to destroy it. It is those who have achieved something and want to rest on their achievements who are forever clogging things up."

And when a chair moves on, he or she should pick the next job carefully. Not every good chair makes a good dean, and clinical chairs, like all leaders, are remembered for the job they botched, especially if the job is their last one. A first-class chair who resigns, becomes a dean, and is inept, will—sadly—be remembered as an inept dean.

# VI

# Looking Back and Looking Forward

## 40
## The Role of Specialization in the Evolution of Clinical Departments

When, about a hundred years ago, clinical departments began evolving into their present form, the chairs of the departments arranged teaching schedules, controlled appointments and promotions, and did all the other things needed to make a department run. The chairs would, I imagine, sometimes seek advice from colleagues, especially from their consultants. But by and large they ran their departments single-handedly.

Then in the 1920s and 1930s, the popularity of this type of organization began to wane (Beeson 1980). Several large departments abandoned the idea of an absolute chair and installed subspecialty units with chiefs. The idea of specialization was not new. Herodotus found specialists in Egypt in the fifth century B.C. "Each physician," he wrote, "is a healer of one disease and no more. All the country is full of physicians, some of the eye, some of the teeth, some of what pertains to the belly, and some of the hidden diagnoses" (1966, 369).

Although the urge to specialize was present in antiquity, there is little evidence that specialization as we know it today played an important role in medicine before the nineteenth century. Kirsner says the first GI clinic was organized in 1885 by Boaz in Berlin. Once the clinic was in operation, Boaz moved quickly. By 1906 he had trained a hundred gastroenterologists and started the first journal in GI disease (1988, 122–23).

While these events were taking place in Germany, the move toward specialization was advancing in the United States and other countries. "Among the most significant of the changes that followed the Franco-Prussian and American Civil Wars," Beeson and Maulitz wrote, "was the segmenting of the medical marketplace, academically and clinically. The process of demarcating new medical specialties, first in Germany and soon after in the other industrial nations, was fueled by two powerful engines: new technology (primarily diagnostic, but also therapeutic) and increased professional competition" (1988, 16).

When, in the late 1800s, the Johns Hopkins Hospital and Medical School opened and ushered in the modern era of medical education in this country, the staff was organized into specialty departments like pathology, medicine, and surgery (Bordley and Harvey 1976, 132–56). And if we define subspecialty divisions as disease-oriented units within specialty departments, we can, I believe, date the beginning of such divisions to the time when William Osler, the first chair of medicine, left Hopkins and Lewellys Barker succeeded him. Barker organized "three research divisions, each with its own laboratory: (1) The Biological Laboratory . . . to concentrate chiefly on infectious diseases. (2) The Physiological Laboratory . . . to be concerned for the most part with cardiovascular and pulmonary diseases. (3) The Chemical Laboratory . . . [which] directed its efforts toward metabolic problems" (267–68). These units were, in a very real sense, the forerunners of our modern-day divisions. And, though it would be years before many departments had such units, their existence at Johns Hopkins heralded a change that would take place in medical schools everywhere.

While these developments were altering the look of medicine in Baltimore, the Hospital of the Rockefeller Institute opened in New

York. The hospital was unique in that, unlike earlier hospitals, it was to be used exclusively for clinical research (Beeson and Maulitz, 21–22). Moreover, the clinical investigators, like professors in clinical departments at Johns Hopkins, would be full time. Being full time was not, of course, the same as being a subspecialist, but the growth of subspecialty divisions, clinical research, and full-time faculty would, in the next few decades, proceed hand-in-hand.

An example of this process may be found in the evolution of the Department of Medicine at the Massachusetts General Hospital. Subspecialization began there in 1920, when J. Howard Means organized a thyroid clinic (Stanbury and Chapman 1983). Two years later, when Means became chair of the Department of Medicine, he added a clinical research unit for patients with thyroid disease. The unit, called Ward 4, had ten beds and its own chemical laboratory. Clinics for other subspecialties, like cardiology, arthritis, and endocrinology, followed. "Over this Hanseatic League of . . . units Means presided benignly and with a loose hand. . . . [although] skilled and devoted physicians filled patient care and teaching responsibilities, there were no organized units or divisions with assigned space for research and postdoctoral training in chest medicine, infectious disease, metabolism, hematology, or allergy-immunology" (Smith and Federman 1983, 70). But when Walter Bauer succeeded Means as the chair of medicine in 1951, he added the missing units and formalized those that already existed. Bauer later described the units in his presidential address to the annual meeting of the Association of American Physicians in 1959. He had, he said, established twelve subspecialty sections, each with its own staff of full- and part-time clinicians and investigators. Each unit resembled "a miniature Departments of Medicine." And such sections, Bauer stressed, needed to be led by chiefs who were competent in basic science as well as in clinical medicine.

"We have," Bauer told his colleagues, "attempted to appoint a particular type of man to head each unit—a man who by some means has managed to plant a solid foot in a scientific discipline beyond the scope of clinical medicine, generally in biochemistry, biophysics, or physiology. . . . By combining clinical medicine and basic science in their training, and by displaying superior competence in both fields, these men represent a new breed of physician" (6).

As these changes were taking place in Boston, the trend toward specialty medicine had been advancing in other parts of the country. By 1927 at the University of Chicago, for example, "gastroenterology under the direction of Walter Lincoln Palmer was a major section within a department of medicine composed entirely of medical specialties" (Kirsner, 122).

At about the same time, a new textbook of medicine gave tacit support to the move toward specialization. Russel Cecil broke with the tradition of single authorship and invited specialists to write parts of his new book. "The rapid growth of medical science during the past few years," Cecil wrote, "has made it almost impossible for a single individual to master the entire field. In internal medicine, as in other branches of human knowledge, the age of specialization has of necessity arrived. [Thus,] it seemed desirable to prepare a textbook of medicine in which each disease, or group of diseases, would be discussed by a writer particularly interested in that subject" (Beeson and Maulitz, 41–42).

Despite these developments, many clinical chairs doubted that specialty divisions were a good idea. William McCann, the distinguished chair of medicine at Rochester was one of the skeptics. Though McCann encouraged the full-time members of the department to develop skill in a subspecialty, they could not divide themselves into divisions, much less have divisional budgets, space, or beds. Categorical groups existed in McCann's department and were "referred to as 'chest lab,' 'hematology lab,' or 'metabolism lab,' " but never as divisions (Beeson 1986, 86). McCann, like other skeptics, believed that all members of clinical departments, even those trained in subspecialties, should—above all else—be generalists.

There were, however, strong opinions on the other side, and W. S. Peart, a member of the medical unit at St. Mary's Hospital in London, crystallized the opinions in the following way: "While fears of super-specialisation in university hospitals, whereby a man may know more and more about less and less, have to be recognised, it is useless to cling to the belief that specialisation can somehow be ignored. It is here, it is expanding, it will bring greater benefits to patients, and it must be contained within a suitable organisation" (1970, 401).

The move toward subspecialties continued in fits and starts through the late 1930s and early 1940s. Then five forces pushed the movement forward with increasing speed.

The ascendancy of the National Institutes of Health was of incalculable importance in this process. Suddenly, the federal government was willing to grant large sums of money to investigators in clinical departments. Equally important, many of the awards were made on a categorical basis—for heart disease, or for cancer, or for some other subspecialty. Hence, it behooved a chair to create groups that could compete for these awards. It was not necessary that the groups be divisions, but divisions were convenient units through which to apply for categorical grants.

The second force promoting specialization, as important as the NIH awards and firmly tied to them, was the slow but steady move toward the creation of full-time faculty positions in clinical departments. In earlier times, community practitioners had taught students and done research in hours stolen from their private practices; but at the turn of the century, as mentioned above, full-time physicians began to appear on clinical faculties—at Johns Hopkins and then at the Hospital of the Rockefeller Institute. By 1950, there were 1,284 full-time faculty members in clinical departments in this country. But in 1976, there would be 33,913 (Siperstein 1980, 1). Departments were becoming so large that their chairs were forced to delegate responsibilities, and divisional chiefs were especially suitable people for these assignments.

A third force moving departments toward chiefs and divisions was the organization of clinics and in-patient services for specific diseases—like the GI clinic in Germany and the thyroid clinic and research ward at the Massachusetts General Hospital. To operate these units, "subspecialists needed to attract colleagues to help with patient care and teaching and to collaborate in research. They wanted to have trainees to assist in consultations around the hospital and to participate in the research. Thus it soon developed that an academic department of medicine was organized in subspecialty divisions" (Beeson and Maulitz, 44). And so were other large academic departments.

A fourth force propelling clinical departments in the direction of subspecialties was the explosion of medical knowledge. The need to specialize, Sir Harold Himsworth asserted in 1955 in his Linacre Lecture, "has arisen because medical knowledge has grown to such an extent that it is no longer, and never again will be, within the capacity of any individual man to master more than a small fraction of it. Specialization has become a necessity. To decry this is not only to ignore facts; it is to deny the very means that have made our recent progress possible. Specialization is a natural phenomenon. It is comparable in human affairs to differentiation of function in biology."

Finally, new drugs and instruments for treating patients, for making diagnoses, and for doing research were proliferating by the month, making mastery of their use by any one person impossible. Even subspecialists had their hands full trying to keep up with advances in their own limited fields.

Under the impetus of these five forces, the trend toward specialization and subspecialty units moved steadily forward. One department after another gave up the idea of an absolute chair and shifted to a chair with chiefs. Now, for large departments, for departments like medicine and surgery, that shift must be virtually complete.

## *41*
## Managed Care

Today, in the waning years of the twentieth century, two words, *managed care*, dominate our thoughts about the practice of medicine. At the moment, these words refer to medical care delivered by health maintenance organizations (HMOs) based in the private sector; but they may come to mean, at some time in the future, care delivered through a global plan run by the government. People like the idea that managed care may reduce the cost of medical coverage, but at the same time they worry that such care will limit their choice of doctors. And physicians worry that managed care may mean mechanized medicine that will, little by little, erode their independence. Meanwhile, HMOs, scattered across the country, are signing up people, physicians, and hospitals at a rapid clip.

Many university hospitals have signed contracts with HMOs, and in these places, clinical chairs have acquired a new set of concerns and problems. One problem has been a drop in the income from clinical practice, because the fee-for-service and capitation payments negotiated by the HMOs have been below those paid by private patients and third party carriers in the past. To offset these reductions, chairs have had to urge department members to see more patients and to process all patients more efficiently.

At the same time, the damage, albeit indirect, that HMOs have done to research programs is of great concern to department chairs. As faculty members have spent more hours seeing patients, they have necessarily had fewer hours for research. Chairs, at the same time, have suffered a loss of flexibility in topping off the partial salaries the researchers get from grants. In the past, chairs were able to piece out these salaries from surplus clinical income, but the tight contracts negotiated by HMOs have sharply reduced a chair's ability to do this.

Some alarmists have said that these reductions in time and flexibility, coupled with dwindling federal funds, may cause clinical departments to revert to the way they were in the early years of this century, when research in clinical departments was the exception, not the rule. And though I said in the chapter on faculty that I doubt anything so drastic will happen, there is no way, at the moment, to refute these dire prophecies, to be certain that the fears are groundless.

Another concern is whether scholarship can flourish in an atmosphere where financial profits have top priority. A. Bartlett Giamatti was skeptical about this (see section 7) and so was Mark van Doren in *Liberal Education* (5). I have no hard data to bring to bear on the question, but I have the same sorts of reservations that Giamatti and Van Doren had. I also have reservations about the effects on scholarship, and on related academic matters, of creating huge departments by the widespread move to consolidate hospitals.

A fourth concern has come from the way managed care may affect the day-to-day practice of medicine. Steve Jones, a young faculty member I know, wrote an essay on what practice is like, these days, in an academic medical center. In describing the shortcomings of the system, Steve had the following things to say about managed care:

> Although the future of managed care is unclear the direction is certain. This new paradigm has both physicians and patients scrambling. Patients must seek out physicians as dictated by their health plans and general finances. Physicians must apply and familiarize themselves with a host of varying managed health plans. Specialists seek now to become generalists. Generalists seek out specialist skills and procedures in order to survive. Uncertainty, anger, frustration, paperwork, paperwork, and more paperwork abound. Oh yes, then there is the patient.
>
> In the outpatient setting, patients are often seen or referred based on their reimbursement potential or managed care plan. Short visits and high volume are encouraged and dictated by financial parameters. The patient's medical needs are usually met, but significant doctor-patient relationships are rare.
>
> Perhaps the most important reform for the future should be the reallotment of time for the physician. Less time caring for charts and

more time caring for patients. Less time managing patient forms and more time managing patient feelings. (1994, 4–5)

Although HMOs have caused the concerns mentioned, they have, at the same time, had beneficial effects. They have reduced the cost of medical coverage, forced hospitals to operate more economically, moved medical practice away from hospital admissions to less expensive ambulatory visits, sometimes brought clinical departments and their associated hospitals closer together, prompted chairs to work cooperatively in designing care-delivery systems, and helped correct a long-talked-about imbalance between general physicians and subspecialists.

Regardless of the way the concerns and benefits settle out, it's useful to remember that this is not the first time a perceived need of society has impinged on a university program. A notable earlier instance came fifty years ago, when World War II threatened liberal education. Events in the early years of the war had forced universities to add courses needed for the war effort, and in making room for these additions, curriculum committees suspended courses in the liberal arts. The suspensions were supposed to be temporary, yet faculty members worried that they might continue after the war ended. Mark van Doren spoke to this worry.

It has long been noted that a circular relation exists between education and society. Each depends on the other to improve it; neither knows whether it is the acorn or the oak. One assumption, however, it has been customary for society to make concerning education: it has its own business to remember, and had better be left free to do it. The mass of men suppose, naively and correctly, that learning keeps a certain distance from life; that universities are places where permanent things are known and the past remains available; that in crises the people should go to the professors, not the professors to the people.

The gravest danger to education now is its own readiness to risk its dignity in a rush to keep up with events, to serve mankind in a low way that will sacrifice respect. The world needs it badly; but so badly that it must study to preserve itself so that it may again be needed and possessed. It can easily prove so useful as to earn contempt. So while it broods upon its own improvement, as it always does, education can afford to ponder programs of being no less deeply than schedules of doing. (5)

In our present state of uncertainty, when our concerns resemble those that plagued Van Doren, I do not, in all truth, worry much about clinical chairs and their departments. During the past hundred years, despite conflicting goals, an explosion of knowledge, six wars, a depression, and three social revolutions, clinical chairs and their departments have survived and flourished. They have carried out their mission marvelously well.

# Appendix

## Bylaws of the Executive Committee of the Department of Medicine of the State University of New York, Stony Brook

1. *Membership.* The executive committee shall consist of:

   a. the director or acting director of the medical service at each clinical campus and each teaching hospital
   b. a staff member designated by the director or acting director of each clinical campus
   c. one professor or one associate professor from each clinical campus and each teaching hospital

   The members mentioned under *c* shall be elected by the medical staff at the campus or hospital, with all staff members holding an appointment of instructor or above being eligible to vote. The elected representative shall: (1) serve for two years, and (2) be ineligible for election to a subsequent term unless one year has elapsed since he or she last held membership.

2. *Functions and Responsibilities.* The executive committee shall be advisory to the chair on all major departmental matters, such as teaching, planning, appointments, and promotions.

3. *Meetings.* Meetings will be held once per three or four weeks, according to a schedule distributed by the chair for each academic year. The schedule shall be mailed to the members in advance of the first meeting.

    The meetings will rotate among the clinical campuses. Emergency meetings can be called at any time by any member by notifying the chair.

    The chair shall preside at each meeting. In his or her absence, the director or acting director at the host clinical campus shall preside.

    A *pro tem* secretary shall be chosen by alphabetical sequence from among the members at the start of each meeting. He or she shall keep minutes, and shall forward a copy to the chair for distribution to all members.

4. *Agendas.* The chair shall distribute copies of the agenda in advance of each meeting. Any member may place a topic for discussion on the agenda by notifying the chair. Emergency matters may be introduced at any meeting without prior notification.

5. *Consultants.* Any member may invite one or more consultants to a meeting by notifying the chair before issuing the invitation.

6. *Amendments to the Bylaws.*

    a. Any member may suggest an amendment at any meeting. Whereas the discussion of the suggested amendment may be concluded at the meeting, or may be carried forward to a subsequent meeting, a vote on the proposal must be delayed until the next meeting after the suggested amendment was introduced. For the vote to take place, fourteen of the nineteen members of the executive committee shall constitute a quorum, provided each campus and teaching hospital has at least one representative present. If these stipulations are fulfilled, the vote of an absent member may be cast by proxy. Approval requires two-thirds of the votes cast.

b. An approved amendment shall be in effect until the annual meeting of the department, when the amendment shall be presented, discussed, approved, or disapproved. Approval shall require 60 percent of the votes cast.

c. Amendments other than those originating in the executive committee can be proposed by any member of the department by: (1) presenting the proposed amendment with a petition signed by 20 percent of the members of the department, (2) requesting that the chair include the proposed amendment in the envelope with the mailing announcing the annual meeting of the department. The procedure for approving the amendment at the annual meeting shall be the same as under 5-b above.

# Bibliography

Adler, M. J., and S. Cain. 1963. *Descartes: Discourse on the Method of Rightly Conducting the Reason.* Vol. 10 of *The Great Ideas Program.* Chicago: Encyclopaedia Britannica.

Adler, M. J., and P. Wolff. 1960. *Foundations of Science and Mathematics.* Vol. 3 of *The Great Ideas Program.* Chicago: Encyclopaedia Britannica.

Aeschylus. 1936. *The Agamemnon of Aeschylus.* Translated by L. MacNeice. London: Faber and Faber.

Allen, T. J. 1970. "Communication Networks in R and D Laboratories." *R and D Management* 1:14–21.

Allen, T. J., and A. R. Fustfeld. 1975. "Research Laboratory Architecture and the Structuring of Communications." *R and D Management* 5:153–164.

*AMA Report of the Citizen's Commission on Graduate Medical Education.* 1966. Chicago: American Medical Association.

Atchley, D. 1964. "The Reminiscences of Dana W. Atchley." *Columbia University Oral History Collection.* Pt. 2, no. 6, p. 108.

Barth, A. 1984. *The Rights of Free Men: An Essential Guide to Civil Liberties.* Edited by J. E. Clayton. New York: Alfred Knopf.

Bartlett, J., ed. 1986. *Familiar Quotations, A Collection of Passages, Phrases and Proverbs Traced to Their Sources in Ancient and Modern Literature.* 14th ed. Boston: Little, Brown.

Bauer, W. 1959. "Medicine in the Teaching Hospital of Today and Tomorrow." *Transactions of the Association of American Physicians* 72:1–10.

Beeson, P. B. 1975. "The Ways of Academic Clinical Medicine in America since World War II." *Men and Medicine* 1:65–79.

Beeson, P. B. 1980. "The Natural History of Medical Subspecialties." *Annals of Internal Medicine* 93:624–626.

Beeson, P. B. 1986. "The Changing Role Model, and the Shift in Power." *Daedalus,* Spring, 83–97.

Beeson, P. B., and R. C. Maulitz. 1988. "The Inner History of Internal Medicine." In *Grand Rounds: One Hundred Years of Internal Medicine*, edited by R. C. Maulitz and D. E. Long. Philadelphia: University of Pennsylvania Press.

Bender, G. A. 1962. "Claude Bernard: Explorer of Physiologic Frontiers." *A History of Medicine in Pictures*. Morris Plains, N.J.: Parke Davis, 1–4.

Bennet, J. B., and D. J. Figuli, eds. 1993. *Enhancing Departmental Leadership: The Role of the Chairperson*. American Council on Education Series on Higher Education. Phoenix, Ariz.: Oryx.

Bergson, H. 1971. *The Creative Mind*. Translated by M. L. Andison. Westport, Conn.: Greenwood.

Bernard, C. 1961. *An Introduction to the Study of Experimental Medicine*. Translated by H. C. Greene. New York: Collier.

Bodin, J. 1958. *Six Books of the Commonwealth*. Abridged and translated by M. J. Tooley. Oxford: Basil Blackwell.

Bordley, J., III, and A. McG. Harvey. 1976. *Two Centuries of American Medicine: 1776–1976*. Philadelphia: W. B. Saunders.

Braunwald, E. 1975. "Can Medical Schools Remain the Optimal Site for the Conduct of Clinical Investigation?" *Journal of Clinical Investigation* 56:i–vi.

Brooks, C. 1985. "What Literature Means in Our Technological Age." *Newsday*, 26 May 1985, sec. "Ideas," 5.

Brown, R. McA. 1955. *The Bible Speaks to You*. Philadelphia: Westminster, 60.

Brumbaugh, R. S. 1962. *Plato for the Modern Age*. New York: Crowell-Collier.

Chesterton, G. K. 1956. *All Things Considered*. New York: Sheed and Ward.

Cohen, I. S. 1962. "Programmed Learning and Socratic Dialogue." *American Psychologist* 17:772–775.

Cowell, A. 1988. "For an Arab, It's the Thought That Counts." *New York Times*, 8 December, C19.

Cutler, P. 1979. *Problem Solving in Clinical Medicine: From Data to Diagnosis*. Baltimore: Williams and Wilkins.

Davis, E. 1954. *But We Were Born Free*. Indianapolis: Bobbs-Merrill.

Deming, W. E. 1982. *Out of the Crisis*. Cambridge: Massachusetts Institute of Technology, Center for Advanced Engineering Study.

Descartes, R. 1910. *Discourse on Method*. Edited by C. W. Eliot. Vol. 34 of *The Harvard Classics*. New York: P. F. Collier and Son.

Drucker, P. F. 1966. *The Effective Executive*. New York: Harper and Row.

Drucker, P. F. 1990. *Managing the Nonprofit Organization: Principles and Practice*. New York: Harper Collins.

Dubos, R. 1986. *Louis Pasteur: Free Lance of Science*. New York: Da Capo.

Eaton, R. P. 1995. "Academic Medical Research: Will Collaboration with Industry and National Laboratories Save It?" *The Pharos*, Fall, 2–4.

Eichna, L. W. 1980. "Medical School Education, 1975–1979: A Student's Perspective." *New England Journal of Medicine* 303:727–734.

Elstein, A. S., L. S. Shulman, and S. A. Sprafka. 1978. *Medical Problem Solving: An Analysis of Clinical Reasoning*. Cambridge: Harvard University Press.

Emrich, J. S. 1992. "Alternative Organizational Structures for the Department of Medicine." In *The Role of the Physician Executive: Cases and Commentary*, edited by D. A. Kindig and A. R. Kovner, 125–147. Ann Arbor: Health Administration Press.

Epstein, J. 1979. *Familiar Territory: Observations on American Life*. New York: Oxford University Press.

Farrar, J. T. 1977. "Franz Joseph Ingelfinger, Master of Maieutics." *American Journal of Digestive Diseases* 22:387–388.

Figuli, D. J. 1993. "Legal Liability: Reducing the Risk." In *Enhancing Departmental Leadership: The Role of the Chairperson*, edited by J. B. Bennet and D. J. Figuli, 141–150. American Council on Higher Education. Phoenix, Ariz.: Oryx.

Finkler, S. A. 1992. *Finance and Accounting for Nonfinancial Managers*. Englewood Cliffs, N.J.: Prentice Hall.

Flesch, R. 1949. *The Art of Readable Writing*. New York: Macmillan.

Flexner, A. 1972. *Medical Education in the United States and Canada, A Report to the Carnegie Foundation for the Advancement of Teaching*. New York: Arno Press and New York Times. Orig. pub. 1910 by D. B. Updike, Merrymount Press, Boston.

Ford, H. 1988. "Points to Ponder." *Reader's Digest*, 19 August, 112.

Fox, A. 1962. "Chapter VII Characteristics." *Plato for Pleasure*. London: John Murray.

Fox-Genovese, E. 1996. "Harassment: The New Weapon of the Gender War." *Newsday*, 27 October, A40–A41.

Freeman, E., and D. Appel. 1956. *The Wisdom and Ideas of Plato.* New York: Fawcett.

Fritts, H. W., Jr. 1977. "Mark Van Doren and the Search for a Rational Curriculum." *The Pharos*, October, 10–12.

Gauss, C. 1980. Introduction to *The Prince*, by N. Machiavelli. Translated by L. Ricci, revised by E. R. P. Vincent. Mentor Edition. New York: New American Library.

Giamatti, A. B. 1988. *A Free and Ordered Space: The Real World of the University.* New York: Norton.

Given, W. R., Jr. 1964. *How to Manage People: The Applied Psychology of Handling Human Problems in Business.* Englewood Cliffs, N.J.: Prentice-Hall.

Glassman, R. B. 1973. Persistence and Loose Coupling in Living Systems. *Behavioral Science* 18:83–98.

Goleman, D. 1991. "Happy or Sad, A Mood Can Prove Contagious." *New York Times*, 15 October, C1.

Greenhouse, L. 1993. "Ginsburg at Fore in Court's Give and Take." *New York Times*, 14 October, A1.

Hamilton, E. 1942. *The Greek Way.* New York: Random House.

Hamilton, L. 1988. "The Campaign: Prose and Cons." *New York Times*, 20 February, Op-Ed.

Hart, M. H. 1987. "René Descartes." *The 100: A Ranking of the Most Influential Persons in History.* Secaucus, N.J.: Citadel, 332–337.

Harvey, A. McG., and J. Bordley. 1970. *Differential Diagnosis: The Interpretation of Clinical Evidence.* Philadelphia: W. B. Saunders.

Harvey, W. P. 1964. "Heart Sounds and Murmurs." *Circulation* 30:262–271.

Haskins, J., and K. Benson. 1988. *The '60s Reader.* New York: Viking Kestral.

Helfand, D. 1986. "I Turned Down Tenure." *Washington Monthly*, June, 13–17.

Henderson, L. J. 1961. Introduction to *An Introduction to the Study of Experimental Medicine*, by Claude Bernard. Translated by H. C. Greene. New York: Collier.

Herodotus. 1966. *Book Two of the Histories.* Translated by A. D. Godley. Loeb Classical Library. Cambridge: Harvard University Press.

Heyssel, R. M., J. R. Gaintner, I. W. Kues, A. A. Jones, and S. H. Lipstein. 1984. "Decentralized Management in a Teaching Hospital." *New England Journal of Medicine* 310:1477–1480.

Himsworth, H. 1955. "The Integration of Medicine: The Endeavour of Thomas Linacre and Its Present Significance." *British Medical Journal* 2:217–222.

Hirschhorn, L. 1995. Leading and Planning in Loosely Coupled Systems (draft). AAMC Executive Development Seminar held October 13–18.

Hoff, H. H., L. Guillemin, and R. Guillemin. 1967. *The Cahier Rouge of Claude Bernard.* Cambridge: Schenkman.

Hoffer, E. 1963. *The Ordeal of Change.* New York: Harper and Row.

Hurst, J. W. 1987. *Notes from a Chairman.* Chicago: Year Book Medical Publishers.

Janis, I. L. 1972. *Victims of Groupthink: A Psychological Study of Foreign-Policy Decisions and Fiascos.* Boston: Houghton Mifflin.

Johns, R. J., N. J. Fortuin, and P. S. Wheeler. 1988. "The Collection and Evaluation of Clinical Information." In *The Principles and Practice of Medicine*, 22nd ed., edited by A. McG. Harvey, R. J. Johns, V. A. McKusick, A. H. Owens, Jr., and R. S. Ross, 4–21. Norwalk, Conn.: Appleton and Lange.

Joint Commission on Accreditation of Healthcare Organizations. 1991. *Using CQI Approaches to Monitor, Evaluate, and Improve Quality.* One Renaissance Drive, Oakbrook Terrace, Illinois 60181.

Jones, S. 1994. "Who's My Doctor?" *Contexts: A Forum for the Medical Humanities* 3:4–5.

Jowett, B., trans. 1937. *Meno.* Vol. 1 of *The Dialogues of Plato.* New York: Random House.

Kassirer, J. P. 1983. "Teaching Clinical Medicine by Iterative Hypothesis Testing: Let's Preach What We Practice." *New England Journal of Medicine* 309:921–923.

Kassirer, J. P., and G. A. Gorry. 1978. "Clinical Problem Solving: A Behavioral Analysis." *Annals of Internal Medicine* 89:245–255.

Kemeny, J. G. 1980. Quoted in "What Is an Educated Person: Three Experts Share Answers." *New York Times*, 18 May, E22.

Kirsner, J. B. 1988. "One Hundred Years of American Gastroenterology." *Grand Rounds: One Hundred Years of Internal Medicine.* Edited by R. C. Maulitz and D. E. Long. Philadelphia: University of Pennsylvania Press.

Klein, J. 1965. *A Commentary on Plato's Meno.* Chapel Hill: University of North Carolina Press.

Kurtz, M. E. 1992. "The Dual Role Dilemma." *The Role of the Physician Executive: Cases and Commentary.* Edited by D. A. Kindig and A. R. Kovner. Ann Arbor: Health Administration Press.

Lasch, C. 1990. "The Lost Art of Political Argument." *Harper's,* September, 17–22.

Levine, R. J., and E. D. Cohen. 1974. "The Hawthorne Effect." *Clinical Research* 22:111–112.

Liebman, J. R. 1946. *Peace of Mind.* New York: Simon and Schuster.

Long, G. 1909. *The Philosophy of Antoninus.* Vol. 2 of *The Harvard Classics.* New York: P. F. Collier and Son.

Machiavelli, N. 1963. *The Prince.* Translated by C. E. Detmold. Edited by L. G. Crocker. New York: Washington Square.

Magee, B. 1973. *Karl Popper.* New York: Viking.

Mahaffy, J. P. 1969. *Descartes.* Freeport, N.Y.: Books for Libraries.

Medawar, P. B. 1990. *The Threat and the Glory: Reflections on Science and Scientists.* New York: Harper Collins.

Metzger, W. P. 1973. "Academic Tenure in America: A Historical Essay." *Faculty Tenure: A Report and Recommendations by the Commission on Academic Tenure in Higher Education.* Edited by W. R. Keast and J. W. Macy, Jr.. San Francisco: Jossey-Bass, 93–159.

Mirvis, D. M., et al. 1994. "Medical School Affiliations with Department of Veterans Affairs Medical Centers: Attitudes of Medical Center Leadership." *American Journal of the Medical Sciences.* 308:162–166.

Montaigne, M. E. de. 1958. *The Complete Essays of Montaigne.* Translated by D. M. Frame. Stanford: Stanford University Press.

Moore, G. E. 1968. *Principia Ethica.* Cambridge: University Printing House.

Newman, J. R. 1956. *The World of Mathematics.* 4 vols. New York: Simon and Schuster.

O'Connor, G. T. 1996. Quoted in "Teamwork Makes Surgeons Better." *Newsday.* 20 March, A60.

O'Connor, G. T. et al. 1996. "A Regional Intervention to Improve the Hospital Mortality Associated with Coronary Artery Bypass Graft Surgery." *Journal of the American Medical Association* 275:841–846.

Olmsted, J. M. D., and E. H. Olmsted. 1952. *Claude Bernard and The Experimental Method in Medicine.* New York: Henry Schuman.

Orton, J. D., and K. E. Weick. 1990. "Loosely Coupled Systems: A Reconceptualization." *Academy of Management Review* 15:203–223.

Osler, W. O. 1947. *Aequanimitas, with Other Addresses to Medical Students, Nurses and Practitioners of Medicine.* 3rd ed. Philadelphia: Blakiston.

Peart, W. S. 1970. "Death of the Professor of Medicine." *Lancet* 1:401–402.

Petersdorf, R. G. 1977. "The President's Address." *Transactions of the Association of American Physicians* 90:1–16.

Petersdorf, R. G. 1984. "The Case against Tenure in Medical Schools." *Journal of the American Medical Association* 251:920–924.

Petersdorf, R. G. 1987. "The VA–Medical School Partnership: The Medical School Perspective." *Journal of Medical Education* 62:153–157.

Petersdorf, R. G. 1991. "If I Had to Do It Again: Suggestions for To-day's Department of Medicine Chairman." *The Pharos*, Winter, 12–16.

Poincaré, H. 1952. *Science and Method.* Translated by F. Maitland. New York: Dover Publications.

Rashkis, H. A., and E. R. Smarr. 1957. "Drug and Milieu Effects with Chronic Schizophrenia." *Archives of Neurology and Psychiatry* 78:89–94.

Richards, D. W. 1962. "Medical Priesthoods, Past and Present." *Transactions of the Association of American Physicians* 75:1–10.

Robinson, J. H. 1921. *The Mind in the Making.* New York: Harper and Brothers.

Rosovsky, H. 1990. *The University: An Owner's Manual.* New York: Norton.

Sarton, G. 1954. *Logan Clendening Lecture on Galen of Pergamon.* Lawrence: University of Kansas Press.

Schlesinger, A. M., Jr. 1993. "Memo to the 1993 Crowd: Believe in Yourselves." *Newsweek*, 11 January, 39.

Schroedinger, E. 1967. *What Is Life?: The Physical Aspect of the Living Cell and Mind and Matter.* Cambridge: Cambridge University Press, 15–17.

Seldes, A., ed. 1985. *The Great Thoughts.* New York: Ballantine.

Selmi, P. M., M. H. Klein, J. H. Greist, S. P. Sorrell, and H. P. Erdman. 1990. "Computer-Administered Cognitive-Behavioral Therapy for Depression." *American Journal of Psychiatry* 147:51–56.

Sigerest, H. E. 1955. *The Great Doctors.* Garden City: Doubleday Anchor.

Siperstein, M. D. 1980. "The Training of Internal Medicine Faculty— 1980." *Transactions of the Association of American Physicians* 93:1–13.

Smith, L. H., Jr., and D. D. Federman. 1983. "Walter Bauer." In *The Massachusetts General Hospital: 1955–1980*, edited by B. Castleman, D. C. Crockett, and S. B. Sutton, 69–76. Boston: Little, Brown.

Smythe, C. McC., A. B. Jones, and M. P. Wilson. 1982. "Tenure in Medical Schools in the 1980s." *Journal of Medical Education* 57:349–360.

Stanbury, J. B., and E. M. Chapman. 1983. "James Howard Means." In *The Massachusetts General Hospital: 1955–1980*, edited by B. Castleman," D. C. Crockett, and S. B. Sutton, 63–68. Boston: Little, Brown.

Tenney, S. M. 1993. "For All Is But a Woven Web of Guesses." *News in Physiological Sciences* 8:51.

Thomas, L. 1979. *The Medusa and the Snail: More Notes of a Biology Watcher.* New York: Viking.

Tucker, A. 1992. "Managing Conflict." In *Chairing the Academic Department.* 3rd ed. New York: American Council on Education and Macmillian Publishing, 397–412.

Tumulty, P. A. 1973. *The Effective Clinician: His Methods and Approach to Diagnosis and Care.* Philadelphia: W. B. Saunders.

Turow, S. 1977. *ONE-L.* New York: G. P. Putnam's Sons.

Van Doren, M. 1959. *Liberal Education.* Boston: Beacon.

Walton, M. 1986. *The Deming Management Method.* New York: Putnam.

Weick, K. E. 1976. "Educational Systems as Loosely Coupled Systems." *Administrative Science Quarterly* 21:1–19.

Weick, K. E. 1982. "Management of Organizational Change among Loosely Coupled Elements." *Changes in Organizations,* edited by P. S. Goodman and Associates. San Francisco: Jossey-Bass.

Winer, L. 1992. "Another Endangered Species." *Newsday,* 8 March, sec. "Fanfare," 5.

Zinsser, W. K. 1988. *Writing to Learn.* New York: Harper and Row.

Zinsser, W. K. 1990. *On Writing Well: An Informal Guide to Writing Nonfiction.* 4th ed. New York: Harper Perennial.

# Index